Roadmap to Recovery

Overcoming Long Haul COVID Syndrome
Accelerate your recovery today
Get your life back

JD GOODMAN

LEGAL NOTICE

The content contained within this book may not be reproduced, duplicated or transmitted without direct written permission from the author or the publisher.

Under no circumstances will any blame or legal responsibility be held against the publisher, or author, for any damages, reparation, or monetary loss due to the information contained within this book.

Either directly or indirectly, you are responsible for your own choices, actions, and results.

This book is copyright protected. This book is only for personal use. You cannot amend, distribute, sell, use, quote or paraphrase any part, or the content within this book, without the consent of the author or publisher.

DISCLAIMER

Please note the information contained within this document is for educational purposes only. All efforts have been made to present accurate, up-to-date, and reliable, complete information.

No warranties of any kind are declared or implied. Readers acknowledge that the author is not engaging in the rendering of legal, financial, medical or professional advice.

The author has no responsibility for the persistence or accuracy of URLs for external or third-party Internet Websites referred to in this publication and does not guarantee that any content on such Websites is, or will remain, accurate or appropriate.

The content within this book has been derived from various sources. Please consult a licensed medical professional before attempting any treatments outlined in this book.

By reading this document, the reader agrees that under no circumstances is the author responsible for any losses, direct or indirect, which are incurred as a result of the use of the information contained within this document, including, but not limited to; errors, omissions, or inaccuracies.

This book is dedicated to all long haul Covid sufferers, their advocacy groups and the front-line doctors and healthcare professionals who are pressing forward with finding treatments for long haul Covid syndrome, using all that medical science and ingenuity can bring forward, to provide relief and find a cure.

INTRODUCTION

Long haul Covid can be considered the next pandemic. Hundreds of thousands of people infected with Covid-19 will suffer debilitating symptoms after recovering from the acute phase.

Mainstream medicine is at a loss as to what causes long haul Covid and how best to treat it.

Their primary treatment protocol is to have interdisciplinary teams of specialists look at the body's different organs exhibiting symptoms. But they don't take a whole-body approach; they don't try to uncover the underlying root causes that might be causing the symptoms associated with long haul Covid, and how it manifests in so many different organs of the body.

Long haul Covid is pushing the frontiers of medicine to move beyond traditional ways of treating disease and examining new ways of understanding a chronic illness such as long haul Covid.

These innovations are helping to usher in creative medical protocols and complementary medical treatments to treat long haul Covid, which go beyond traditional approaches and utilize a wider field of health science to foster recovery.

This roadmap will identify and present research that underlies many of these new treatments. It asks what would a person suffering from long haul Covid need or want to know? What would be helpful to them? What are some potential solutions?

It will inform readers of the many new treatment methods used to bring about the alleviation of symptoms, recovery, and gaining your life back.

The longer sufferers wait to treat symptoms, the longer it will take to recover.

With the knowledge presented here, readers can hopefully accelerate their recovery and return to everyday life as quickly as possible.

TABLE OF CONTENTS

TABLE OF CONTENTS

01

Long Haul Covid

Chapter One
About the Syndrome & How Long It Lasts

KEY FACTS

- Most Covid-19 patients recover within weeks
- Covid-19 symptoms can return months after a negative test
- Can result in a wide range of symptoms that last for months
- Has a variety of names
- Three types: Long Covid, Multi-Organ or Auto-Immune, Effects of Hospitalization
- Mental health issues after Covid-19

Covid-19 is an infectious disease caused by the SARS-CoV-2 virus. Among the family of coronavirus diseases, Covid-19 causes acute respiratory tract infections in humans that last approximately two weeks in mild or moderate cases.

Symptoms can persist for months causing damage to the lungs, heart, liver, kidneys, nervous system, and other major organs.[1] But many patients who had mild symptoms from which they recovered reported experiencing lingering health problems following the acute phase of the illness, including heart palpitations, brain fog, cardiovascular strain, and other symptoms long after their recovery.

Grief, loss, fatigue and post-traumatic stress are all mental health effects that can also result from the treatment and recovery from Covid-19.

The Centres for Disease Control and Prevention (CDC) reports that although most people with Covid-19 get better within weeks of illness, some do not. Even people who do not require hospitalization and have mild illnesses can experience persistent symptoms or long-term effects.

Older patients and those with underlying health conditions are at increased risk for the severe disease at the time of infection and later having long-term effects.

However, even young people without underlying health conditions have reported long-lasting symptoms and conditions after the initial disease, including those with asymptomatic infection. It's also important to note a wide range of post-Covid conditions with varying health effects. Post-Covid disorders are characterized by the development and persistence of new or recurrent symptoms after the acute illness has resolved.[2]

The CDC says that people commonly report different combinations of the following symptoms:[3]

- Difficulty breathing or shortness of breath
- Tiredness or fatigue
- Symptoms that get worse after physical or mental activities
- Difficulty thinking or concentrating (sometimes referred to as "brain fog")
- Cough
- Chest or stomach pain
- Headache
- Fast-beating or pounding heart (also known as heart palpitations)
- Joint or muscle pain
- Pins-and-needles feeling
- Diarrhea
- Sleep problems

- Fever
- Dizziness on standing (light-headedness)
- Rash
- Mood changes
- Change in smell or taste
- Changes in period cycles

According to the CDC, some people experience a range of new or ongoing symptoms that can last weeks or months after being infected with the virus that causes Covid-19.

Unlike some other types of post-Covid conditions that only tend to occur in people who have had a severe illness, these symptoms can happen to anyone who has had Covid-19, even if the disease was mild or had no initial symptoms.[4]

Long haul Covid symptoms have been compared to other conditions, such as myalgic encephalomyelitis/ chronic fatigue syndrome (ME/CFS), dysautonomia or postural orthostatic tachycardia syndrome (POTS), mast cell activation syndrome (MCAS), Multisystem Inflammatory Syndrome in Children (MIS-C) and Pediatric Autoimmune Neuropsychiatric Disorders Associated with Streptococcal Infections (PANDAS).[5]

A study published in the Lancet concurred with these results, adding post-treatment Lyme disease to the list.[6]

The CDC refers to post-Covid conditions by a wide range of names, including "post-acute Covid-19," "long-term effects of Covid," "long Covid," "post-acute Covid syndrome," "chronic Covid," "long haul Covid," "late sequelae," and others; as well as the research term used by the National Institutes of Health (NIH): post-acute sequelae of SARS-CoV-2 infection (PASC).[7]

A clinical study published by The Lancet reports that there were more than 200 symptoms associated with long haul Covid sufferers. Memory loss, hallucinations, tremors, fatigue, and many other serious illnesses were attributed to patients long after their recovery from the disease.

The study included 4,000 participants from 56 countries who identified fatigue, brain fog and physical or mental malaise among the most common symptoms.[8]

FAIR Health reports that pain was the most common symptom, followed by shortness of breath, high levels of triglycerides, fatigue, hypertension, anxiety, intestinal issues, skin issues, high blood sugar, cholesterol or blood pressure and abnormal heart results.[9]

The study published in the scientific magazine Nature reports that beyond the first 30 days of illness, people with Covid-19 are at higher risk of death and more likely to exhibit nervous system and neurocognitive disorders, mental health disorders, metabolic disorders, cardiovascular disorders and gastrointestinal disorders.

The study found that these outcomes were just as likely for patients not requiring hospitalization for the acute phase of infection as those who were hospitalized.[10]

CDC has classified three general types of post-Covid conditions: long Covid, multi-organ or autoimmune, and effects of hospitalization. The categories are not mutually exclusive as people can have multiple types of effects across the spectrum.

The first, called long Covid, involves a range of symptoms that can last for months after first being infected with SARS-CoV-2 or can even first appear weeks after the acute phase of infection has resolved.

Even if the illness was mild or entirely asymptomatic, long-Covid could happen to anyone infected with SARS-CoV-2.

People with long Covid report experiencing varied symptoms, including tiredness or fatigue, abnormal sleep patterns, difficulty thinking or concentrating (sometimes referred to as "brain fog"), headache, loss of smell or taste, fast-beating or pounding heart (also known as heart palpitations), chest pain, shortness of breath, cough, joint or muscle pain, depression, anxiety, and fever.

The causes of long Covid are still unclear, although there are several hypotheses, including damage to blood vessels, autoimmune effects, and ongoing infection.[11]

Multiorgan effects of Covid-19 are the second type of post-Covid condition as described on CDC's website. Covid-19 can affect and cause long-term damage in multiple organ systems, including those involving the heart, lung, kidney, and brain. These effects can include conditions that occur shortly after the acute phase of SARS-CoV-2 infection, like multisystem inflammatory syndrome (MIS) and autoimmune disorders.

MIS is a condition where different body parts can become inflamed. CDC is studying inflammatory symptoms in both children (called MIS-C) and adults (called MIS-A). Covid-19 illness can also precede the development of autoimmune responses, which cause the immune system to attack healthy cells by mistake and damage different parts of the body. Multiorgan effects include neurological conditions, kidney damage or failure, diabetes, cardiovascular damage, and skin conditions.[12]

In the final category, post-Covid conditions also include the longer-term effects of Covid-19 treatment or hospitalization. Some of these longer-term effects for hospitalized patients are like those seen in people hospitalized for other reasons, such as severe respiratory infections caused by different viruses or bacteria.

Effects of Covid-19 treatment and hospitalization include post-intensive care syndrome, which refers to health effects that remain after a critical illness. Post-intensive care syndrome has severe weakness, brain dysfunction, and mental health problems like stress disorders. Some of these symptoms can overlap with those observed with long Covid.[13]

7

According to Johns Hopkins University, there are many linkages to be made between Covid-19 and a wide range of symptoms in long haulers. Permanent scarring of the lungs can cause persistent shortness of breath with the result that it could take months for lung function to return to normal if at all, requiring patients to engage in respiratory therapy.

Heart problems were reported in 60% of post-Covid patients, including heart inflammation, palpitations, and rapid heartbeat. Where the initial infection caused damage to the kidneys, long-term kidney disease can result in the need for dialysis.

Senses of smell or taste are often affected by Covid-19 and can cause loss of appetite, anxiety, and depression, with most issues resolving within a year for most post-Covid patients. Neurological problems such as brain fog, headache, fatigue, and dizziness and other neurocognitive symptoms can persist for up to a year following infection.

Diabetes, especially type 2, is a risk factor in serious cases of Covid-19 infection and some post-Covid patients have reported developing type 2 diabetes. The autonomic nervous system is also affected by Covid-19, with post-Covid patients experiencing problems with blood circulation.[14]

The Mayo Clinic reports that the experiences of Covid-19 survivors make them more likely to develop mood disorders, including post-traumatic stress syndrome, depression, and anxiety.

This is especially relevant to hospitalized patients who spent time being treated in intensive care and required the use of mechanical ventilators. Many people who recovered from severe acute respiratory syndrome (SARS) went on to develop chronic fatigue syndrome, a disorder that causes extreme physical and mental fatigue.[15]

Johns Hopkins University says that some survivors of Covid-19 suffer anxiety, depression, and other mental health issues. Pain, weakness, loss of good health, periods of isolation, stress from job loss or financial difficulties, grief from the death of loved ones are all experiences that can affect patients' mental health.

Prolonged periods spent in intensive care can cause lasting and recurrent feelings of terror or dread, including post-traumatic stress disorder.

Some patients have reported experiencing hallucinations and delirium.[16] A study published in the Journal of Gerontology that included 4,900 older adults hospitalized due to Covid-19 says that 11% of patients experienced altered mental status.[17]

Chapter Two
Who Gets Long Haul Covid

KEY FACTS

- One in four patients regardless of the severity
- No clear link between risk factors
- Those with COVID-19 who are hospitalized and those who have a mild illness
- Older patients with co-morbidities are at increased risk
- Asymptomatic patients are at risk
- Young patients without underlying conditions

The prevalence of long haul Covid in the population is more common than most people think and those at risk of developing symptoms encompass a much wider segment of the post-Covid patients.

UC Davis Health reports that long haul Covid afflicts twenty-five per cent of patients regardless of the severity of their infection or other risk factors such as age or health history. This finding applied to non-hospitalized patients and even asymptomatic patients.[18]

NBC News reports that approximately 8.4 million Americans are afflicted with long haul Covid with more than eighty "post-Covid" clinics across the nation specializing in the treatment of patients of all ages with lingering symptoms.[19]

One US study reported that only 65% of patients returned to previous levels of health two to three weeks following the onset of infection.[20]

Johns Hopkins University says that while it's clear that people with certain risk factors (including high blood pressure, smoking, diabetes, obesity, and other conditions) are more likely to have a severe bout of Covid-19, there isn't a clear link between these risk factors and long-term problems. Long haul Covid can happen in people who have mild symptoms.[21]

The Mayo Clinic reports that older people with underlying medical conditions are more likely to develop "lingering Covid-19 symptoms," while admitting that young, healthy people can feel unwell for weeks and months following infection.[22]

They also report that though the disease primarily infects the lungs, there is evidence of further damage to the heart and brain. Imaging tests taken months after recovery from Covid-19 have shown lasting damage to the heart muscle.

The type of pneumonia often associated with Covid-19 can cause long-standing damage to the tiny air sacs (alveoli) in the lungs. There is even the risk of long-lasting damage to the brain, including strokes, seizures, and Guillain-Barre syndrome.[23]

According to the Public Health Agency of Canada, eight in ten people had at least one long-term symptom at least four to twelve weeks following diagnosis, with more than half reporting symptoms after twelve weeks. Reported symptoms included fatigue, pain, shortness of breath, sleep disturbance, anxiety, cough, and hair loss.[24]

FAIR Health reports that at least 19% of patients exhibited at least one post-Covid condition thirty days following an initial Covid-19 diagnosis.

FAIR Health's database of nearly two million Covid-19 patients, the largest population of Covid-19 patients ever studied, confirmed post-Covid symptoms were more common following severe cases, approximately half of cases.

Yet, 27.5% of non-hospitalized patients later presented new health issues, and 19% of asymptomatic patients sought medical attention thirty days following an initial positive test.

The odds of death 30 days or more after a Covid-19 infection was 46 times higher for those hospitalized and discharged than for non-hospitalized people.[25]

The young are not immune to long haul Covid symptoms. The CDC reports that while it is very rare, some people, mostly children, experience multisystem inflammatory syndrome (MIS) during or immediately after a Covid-19 infection.

MIS is a condition where different body parts can become inflamed. MIS can lead to post-Covid conditions if a person continues to experience multiorgan effects or other symptoms.[26]

Johns Hopkins University reports that some young Covid-19 patients experience the rare complication of the multisystem inflammatory syndrome in children, or MIS-C, which can cause serious heart damage requiring a pediatric cardiologist.

They say that though it is not yet known if children who experience Covid-19 are more or less likely to experience long haul symptoms, they are known to exhibit the same symptoms as adults with long Covid symptoms.[27]

Chapter Three
How Long Haul Covid Is Challenging the Healthcare System

KEY FACTS

- It is the next public health disaster in the making
- Disability costs could become catastrophic
- Current medical guidelines fail to adequately account for long haul Covid patients
- The rigid medical system not set up to handle an influx of such diverse patients
- Poised to join other post-infectious syndromes (e.g., fibromyalgia, Lyme disease, etc)
- Lessons of dysautonomia sufferers
- Long hauler support groups will become key to navigating the system

Multiple sources warn that long haul Covid presents serious challenges to the integrity of the healthcare system and risks becoming the next public health disaster following a pandemic that has already caused so much devastation.

Johns Hopkins University points out that the sheer scale of patients with Covid-19 is difficult and that post-viral symptoms and diseases pose a wider challenge to the healthcare system.

As evidenced by post-viral sufferers of previous outbreaks such as SARS (severe acute respiratory syndrome) or MERS (Middle East respiratory syndrome), the potential of health problems in patients who recover from the disease following the epidemic or pandemic creates new pressures upon healthcare providers.[28]

In an article published in The Atlantic, Craig Spencer, Director of Global Health in Emergency Medicine at New York-Presbyterian/Columbia University Irving Medical Centre offers sobering words. "What people need to know is the pandemic's toll is likely much higher than we are imagining. It is an area that merits urgent attention. There will be people living with the impact of Covid long after the pandemic is over."[29]

The CDC reports that post-Covid conditions also include the longer-term effects of Covid-19 treatment or hospitalization. Some of these longer-term effects for hospitalized patients are like those seen in people hospitalized for other reasons, such as severe respiratory infections caused by different viruses or bacteria.[30]

The CDC admits that some symptoms that can occur after hospitalization are like some of the signs that people with initially mild or no symptoms may experience many weeks after Covid-19. It can be challenging to know whether they are caused by the effects of hospitalization, the long-term effects of the virus, or a combination of both.

These conditions might also be complicated by other effects of the Covid-19 pandemic, including mental health effects from isolation, negative economic situations, and lack of access to healthcare for managing underlying conditions. These factors have affected both people who have experienced Covid-19 and those who have not.[31]

The New England Journal of Medicine calls long Covid "the next public health disaster in the making." They argue that the multispecialty, organ-focused health care system in the United States is not set up to deal with long Covid patients.

Part of the problem is that there is no universal definition of the condition nor are there currently accepted objective diagnostic tests or biomarkers.

The average age of long Covid patients is around 40, meaning many of these working-age patients are more likely to need access to various disability supports and programs.[32]

Historical precedents of similar post-infection syndromes such as myalgic encephalomyelitis/chronic fatigue syndrome (ME/CFS), fibromyalgia, and post-treatment Lyme disease syndrome demonstrate the lasting challenges of diagnosis and treatment presented by these complex diseases.

In many cases, the medical community is slow to recognize these syndromes, forcing patients into circuitous pathways to recovery. The costs of these unrecognized illnesses not yet considered legitimate by the medical community are thus externalized onto society. Patients feel misunderstood, even disbelieved, by their doctors.[33]

The same New England Journal of Medicine report emphasized the scale of the problem, as 40 million Americans infected with Covid-19 translate to a conservative estimate of 15 million long Covid cases resulting from the pandemic.[34]

These conditions are favourable for the development of support groups. The Body Politic Covid-19 Support Group already has 25,000 members and others are popping up across the US. In Britain, one group, called LongCovidSOS, lobbied the government to recognize long Covid and push for research and support systems.

Such groups have formed alliances with other groups such as myalgic encephalomyelitis and dysautonomia sufferers, turning to one another when the medical establishment failed to adequately recognize their needs.[35]

The Cleveland Clinic reports that dysautonomia, or autonomic neuropathy, is an umbrella term for various conditions that share the common problem of an autonomic nervous system (ANS) that doesn't function normally.

The ANS controls involuntary body functions such as heart rate, blood pressure, breathing, digestion, body and skin temperature, hormonal, bladder, sexual and other functions.

An ANS disorder can cause a host of problems that may be diagnosed as its disorder or secondary to various other diseases such as Parkinson's, muscular sclerosis, lupus, sarcoidosis, Crohn's, amyloidosis, or Lyme disease among others.

The syndrome is shared by some 70 million people worldwide and can be either congenital or acquired. Given that symptoms vary widely from patient to patient, it can be considered analogous to the situation faced by long haul Covid sufferers.[36]

As above, many long haul Covid sufferers have experienced problems with their autonomic nervous system. The Atlantic reports that some theories speculate long Covid results from a powerful immune reaction to the virus which results in widespread damage to the body which may cause autoimmune diseases. Others posit that the virus causes direct damage to the nervous system.[37]

Given the similarly wide range of experiences of those experiencing long Covid, many of them may join the ranks of millions of dysautonomia sufferers before theirs is recognized as its own syndrome.

According to the Scientific American, a major policy and planning gap awaits U.S. policymakers. Unlike the common cold or flu, post-Covid patients present a range of symptoms that persist long after the initial illness and do not resume their usual activities. Policymakers and planners are urged to consider the long-term consequences and prepare for millions of people likely seeking to draw upon worker's compensation, disability insurance programs and support services.

Many sufferers have already reported they are unable to return to work months after their initial illness, and there are untold millions who may enter the ranks of the permanently disabled.

"How many 'long haulers' will never be able to return to work? How many will need short-term disability payments? How many will be permanently disabled and become dependent on disability programs? As increasing numbers of younger people become infected, will we see an entire generation of chronically ill?"

Health care costs may skyrocket as people lose or are reduced to precarious jobs. The strain on worker's compensation and disability support systems could reach a breaking point. Current disability programs are underequipped to deal with the coming problem of post-Covid patients and the bureaucracy of existing silos of disability support, such as worker's compensation, Social Security disability, and private disability insurance.[38]

Chapter Four
Eight Months of Long Covid Brought Me to The Brink

Opinion by Morgan Stephens
Updated 10:56 AM ET, Fri July 23, 2021

Morgan Stephens is a journalist living and working in Los Angeles and a production assistant for CNN's "Erin Burnett OutFront." Her writing has appeared in CNN Politics and Huffpost. She covered the Trump administration in 2019 with the CBS News White House unit as an intern. Follow her on Twitter. The opinions expressed in this commentary are her own. View more opinion on CNN.

(CNN) As Americans continue to become infected with the new highly contagious Delta variant of the coronavirus -- and every US state and Washington DC sees a rise in Covid-19 cases, about 10%, doctors say, will go on to develop what I've been struggling with for months: long Covid-19 — or lingering symptoms post-infection that are difficult to diagnose.

Both my experience and the stories I've heard of many Americans continuing to deal with the mental and physical anguish that comes from being a long hauler should motivate Congress to support bi-partisan initiatives like the COVID-19 Long Haulers Act, which died in the last congressional session but was reintroduced this year. Covid-19 will continue to cause havoc until more Americans get vaccinated.

For me, the ordeal started in November, four weeks after I'd contracted Covid, two weeks after I was no longer testing positive and months before vaccines were widely available in the US. My body shook for five days before I checked myself into a North Carolina hospital. A surge of adrenaline coursed through me as I slogged through the packed waiting room and curled up on a linoleum bench to wait for someone to tell me what was wrong.

Two nights earlier, what felt like a brain zap jolted me awake. I staggered into the hallway on a funhouse tilt. My world, a Salvador Dali painting, distorted and oozing. Speak, I told myself, but the words came out drowsy and slow.

Only a year before, I was reporting on the Iowa caucus, gaggling with presidential candidates, interning with the White House press corps and becoming the first in my family to graduate from college -- at the top of my class. Despite taking precautions, my mother, father, husband and I contracted Covid-19 in November, six months after I landed a job at CNN.

Unlike many of the 181 million, globally, who survived coronavirus, I did not get better and my life did not return to "normal." In fact, what came next was much worse, even if it can't be detected by tests. One month later and I was in the emergency room. "Your blood work looks great," the doctor said.

"I have this shaky, electric feeling in my stomach," I said. "I can't think. I can't sleep." The doctor asked if I had seen the latest "60 Minutes" with Anderson Cooper on "long haulers." "I've seen it. I work in news."

I had been producing coverage of post-Covid-19 symptoms with the "Erin Burnett OutFront" team. I had watched the episode, thinking this was only something that happened to other people. What others described in our interviews came to mind: "tremors," "brain fog," "paralysis."

She told me I was the third person she'd seen with this. The others landed in her emergency room two and three months post-infection. I was four weeks in from my initial infection.

The doctor handed me my medical papers and discharged me: 30-year-old female. Post-acute Covid syndrome. "Watch that episode," she advised, then left. I started to cry.

The tremors and vertigo had intensified. It'd been a week without sleep. And, with no medical treatment, I was essentially charged thousands for an emergency room visit and given a prescription for Anderson Cooper.

When it came to long Covid-19, even in America's hospitals, there were no experts to be found.

A recent FAIR Health study of Covid-19 patients -- the largest to date, analyzing the health records of nearly two million people who have been infected with the virus in the US found that hundreds of thousands have sought care for new health conditions after their acute illness subsided.

If our illnesses extend for more than a year, we'll need to file for federal disability through the Social Security Administration. More businesses will need to pay sick employees and the US health care system -- which has health care workers leaving or considering leaving the profession altogether -- will continue to be stretched beyond its limits. More congressional funding should go to efforts that are monitoring illnesses associated with long Covid.

Since December, I've seen 15 specialists, received eight scans, visited three ERs and -- even with insurance -- spent $12,000 seeking a return to normal life. Since February, I moved across the country to receive treatment from a post-Covid recovery clinic at my alma mater, Keck School of Medicine of University of Southern California. The clinic refers its patients to specialists depending on their symptoms and provides a social worker.

I receive weekly treatment from a physical therapist, occupational therapist and neurologist there.

Other than the vague "post-acute Covid syndrome," a term that shows up more than 100 million times in Google searches, I've been given no diagnosis. This might be because clinical guidance for physicians has yet to come.

I've had more than 50 symptoms ranging from cognitive impairment, insomnia, vertigo, extreme light and sound sensitivity, and fatigue to convulsion-like shaking, slurred speech, hair loss, muscle weakness, anxiety. The majority occurred simultaneously. The ability to write marks a significant improvement; for six months I couldn't do it. Still, I haven't had a symptom-free day since November 6, 2020, the day I tested positive for Covid-19.

One of the most sinister things about long Covid-19 is its ability to hide from testing. The very nature of our syndrome compels us to question ourselves ad nauseam until we capitulate in exhaustion. *OK, then why can't I walk without panting? Why can't I follow along in conversations even though listening is what I do for a living?*

The mental gymnastics I went through each time the cage cha-chinked shut around my head for an MRI or a technician tacked electrodes to my head for an EEG was exhausting. I was terrified of something showing up, yet I desperately wanted proof because with proof there might be a solution. But nothing abnormal ever showed.

Drowning in Fog

In the early months, existence shrunk to survival. I was too foggy to read. I stopped watching TV, including the very news that I had worked years to be a part of. I stopped communicating with the outside world and deleted my social media accounts -- they were too painful to look at. In dreams, I fell into large bodies of water trapped inside a car. It wasn't until I heard discussions -- Wait, a group stormed the Capitol? Donald Trump got impeached again? -- that I stumbled through the ritual of eating. Pick up the orange. Lift, chew, set it down.

Mental health care for long haulers also cannot be a side note. The deaths of Texas Roadhouse CEO Kent Taylor and "Dawson's Creek" writer Heidi Ferrer revealed the heightened risk of suicide long Covid brings.

"Long haulers need immediate access -- which they're not getting -- to mental health care and a national fund to deal with issues caused by long Covid," Ferrer's husband Nick Guthe told me. "We need a bridge until research can catch up."

I debated with myself whether to share details about my darkest moments. Often journalists may not feel comfortable sharing their struggles with mental health: stoicism can feel all but required when your job is to field tragedies daily. Some may feel it makes them look weak, or unreliable, or could be held against them. Without it, though, I wouldn't be telling the full story.

Before my illness, I never had any thoughts about suicide. This changed after I got sick. I'm no longer in this dark place, but the months it held me hostage I inched closer to the edge than I ever wished to be.

As my brain fog intensified, I developed such a palpable anxiety, it brought with it new compulsive behaviors like "trichotillomania," or hair pulling.

The days blended into one dream-state. I had only what I can describe as brain zaps. I'd wash my hair, forget, then wash it again. The further I slipped away from reality, the deeper my depression became.

I found myself researching death-with-dignity laws. I learned that Northern European countries have some of the most lenient.

Afternoons were filled with anguish. For weeks I'd throw myself on the floor, writhe there and bury my face into the living room rug. Maybe if I lay here long enough I'll free myself from my body.

My mother had been trying her best to keep me above water, but my illness webbed out, becoming more oppressive as the weeks rolled on — when we acknowledged I wasn't getting better. Each day she sat with me in silence.

Each night, she was my partner in pain. In the mornings, she brewed tea, prepared a plate of berries, toast and yogurt that she'd prod me to eat. She quietly went through each room, removing the clocks on the wall after I casually mentioned their ticking made me jump. In the afternoons she sat patiently over the bathtub running her hands under the spout, dropping bits of lavender oil into the water. Then, she'd peel me from the mattress and I'd stagger in.

It was gut-wrenching to watch my family desperately search for answers and after most visits, becoming just as disappointed when the response from medical health professionals was "We just don't know enough about Covid-19 yet to help."

Long Covid is not the typical medical crisis but a slow burn of an illness -- something emergency medicine has little use for.

The abrupt deterioration of my mental health from this is not unique. Many on Body Politic, an online support group for long haulers that's helped me, shared that they, too, had thoughts of ending their life.

"I'm against suicide but I told my partner to hide our gun from me," Angela, a mother of two young children who asked to keep her last name anonymous, told me in January. "I didn't trust knowing where it was."

Research and mental health care lags behind patient experience

Science is catching up, slowly -- but it needs time. Research is pointing to neuropsychiatric changes in Covid-19 survivors potentially due to inflammation or a disruption of blood flow to the brain. There are theories that the virus affects serotonin and dopamine neurotransmitters. According to a study at Oxford, Covid-19 may change the physiology of the brain. A recent case published in the Journal of Psychiatry Neuroscience and Therapeutics reported "autoimmune-mediated psychosis" after a 30-year-old without previous health conditions developed delusions.

But we need more.

It was a two-month wait to see a psychiatrist. This is unacceptable. Having access to psychiatrists and psychologists is critical to recovery. And when we're seen, approaching long Covid with the conventional assessments historically seen as "hysteria," or slapping on a psychiatric diagnosis without considering broader multi-system involvement is what will keep long-haulers sicker, longer.

That's not to say chronic illness doesn't cause psychological distress like post-traumatic stress disorder (PTSD) and depression, but experts must be aware of the constellation of post-Covid symptoms -- there are many and the challenge isn't easy -- then assess from that starting point.

Discussions with long haulers often end in, "I've given up on doctors," or "I'm just glad to be alive," or even sometimes on a bad day, an exasperated, "I'm so fu**ing tired of this."

We're the first of our kind. We're bound together in our collective trauma -- the one that's been invisible to others. And our numbers are growing.

Today, I still experience severe vertigo, fatigue, brain fog, exercise intolerance, screen sensitivity, insomnia and migraines.

I think of the night before Christmas -- the night I surrendered after, at that point, dealing with these mysterious symptoms for four weeks. The night I assumed that whatever was wrong with me was probably going to kill me.

I sat hurriedly scribbling out notes to my family. The smell of cinnamon and lilies from the get-well bouquet my "OutFront" team sent filled the room. Hmph, I can smell again, I thought as I feverishly tried to form the sentences that my family would read. Putting thoughts into words was like wading through molasses.

I just couldn't do it. So, I plainly thanked my mother, father and husband -- and I planned. I wrote that I wanted my body to be donated to science. It haunts me to know that, at that moment, I was still worried about being missed as a Covid-related death.

Yes, I'm glad to be alive too, but I want more for us. With support from our health care providers and policymakers, I want those living in the shadows of long Covid to come out of a dark winter and heal in the sun.

If you are struggling with depression and suicidal thoughts, please call the National Suicide Prevention Lifeline at 1-800-273-8255. The International Association for Suicide Prevention and Befrienders Worldwide also can provide contact information for crisis centers around the world.

Courtesy CNN

PART TWO

02

How We Got Here

Chapter Five
Where We Are Now

KEY FACTS

- A highly contagious virus that has spread across the globe since 2019
- Delta variant more transmissible than the original virus
- The virus spreads through aerosolized particles inhaled or touched
- Upwards of 223 million cases worldwide, more than 4.6 million deaths
- Seniors and immunocompromised individuals are most, but not solely, at risk
- Vaccines effective against severe disease and death
- Patients infected with Covid-19 developed lasting immunity

Covid-19 or SARS-CoV-2 was first identified in Wuhan, China on December 31, 2019. It is highly contagious and has since spread across the globe. On March 11, 2020 the World Health Organization (WHO) declared the Covid-19 outbreak a global pandemic.

The WHO reports that as of September 10, 2021, there have been more than 223 million cases worldwide and 4.6 million confirmed deaths. In the United States, the CDC reports almost 41 million cases and more than 654 thousand deaths.

In addition, there have been more than 1.5 million cases and slightly more than 27 thousand deaths in Canada, and the European Centre for Disease Prevention and Control reported nearly 40 million cases and 759 thousand deaths.

Public health officials warn that the elderly and immunocompromised people are most at risk, yet youth are also at risk.

The National Center for Health Statistics reports that as of August 18, 2021, 361 children died from Covid-19. Deaths of patients in the age category 0-24 are tracked by comorbidities such as respiratory illness, pneumonia, obesity, circulatory system diseases and sepsis.[39]

According to a meta-analysis study published in the International Journal of Infectious Diseases, of 42 studies containing 275,661 children without comorbidities and 9,353 children with comorbidities, severe COVID-19 was present in 5.1% of children with comorbidities, and in 0.2% without comorbidities.[40]

According to the CDC, the principal mode by which people are infected with SARS-CoV-2 (the virus that causes Covid-19) is through exposure to respiratory fluids carrying the infectious virus.

Exposure occurs in three principal ways: (1) inhalation of very fine respiratory droplets and aerosol particles, (2) deposition of respiratory droplets and particles on exposed mucous membranes in the mouth, nose, or eye by direct splashes and sprays, and (3) touching mucous membranes with hands that have been soiled either directly by virus-containing respiratory fluids or indirectly by touching surfaces with the virus on them.[41]

People release respiratory fluids during exhalation (e.g., quiet breathing, speaking, singing, exercise, coughing, sneezing) in the form of droplets across a spectrum of sizes. These droplets carry the virus and transmit infection.

- The largest droplets settle out of the air rapidly, within seconds to minutes.
- The smallest very fine droplets, and aerosol particles formed when these fine droplets rapidly dry, are small enough that they can remain suspended in the air for minutes to hours.

Infectious exposures to respiratory fluids carrying SARS-CoV-2 occur in three principal ways (not mutually exclusive):

1. **Inhalation** of air carrying very small fine droplets and aerosol particles that contain the infectious virus. The risk of transmission is greatest within three to six feet of an infectious source where the concentration of these very fine droplets and particles is greatest.
2. **Deposition** of virus carried in exhaled droplets and particles onto exposed mucous membranes (i.e., "splashes and sprays", such as being coughed on). The risk of transmission is likewise greatest close to an infectious source where the concentration of these exhaled droplets and particles is greatest.
3. **Touching** mucous membranes with hands soiled by exhaled respiratory fluids containing a virus or from touching inanimate surfaces contaminated with the virus.[42]

The risk of SARS-CoV-2 infection varies according to the amount of virus to which a person is exposed.

The CDC says with increasing distance from the source, the likelihood of infection through inhalation likewise decreases.

Although infections through inhalation at distances greater than six feet from an infectious source are less likely than at closer distances, the phenomenon has been repeatedly documented under certain preventable circumstances.

These transmission events have involved the presence of an infectious person exhaling virus indoors for an extended time (more than 15 minutes and in some cases hours) leading to virus concentrations in the air space sufficient to transmit infections to people more than 6 feet away, and in some cases to people who have passed through that space soon after the infectious person left.

Per published reports, factors that increase the risk of SARS-CoV-2 infection under these circumstances include:

- **Enclosed spaces with inadequate ventilation or air handling** within which the concentration of exhaled respiratory fluids, especially very fine droplets and aerosol particles, can build up in the air space.
- **Increased exhalation** of respiratory fluids if the infectious person is engaged in physical exertion or raises their voice (e.g., exercising, shouting, singing).
- **Prolonged exposure** to these conditions, typically more than 15 minutes.[43]

Once infectious droplets and particles are exhaled, they move outward from the source. The risk for infection decreases with increasing distance from the source and increasing time after exhalation. Two principal processes determine the amount of virus to which a person is exposed in the air or by touching a surface contaminated by virus:

1. **The decreasing concentration of virus in the air** as larger and heavier respiratory droplets containing virus fall to the ground or other surfaces under the force of gravity and the very fine droplets and aerosol particles that remain in the airstream progressively mix with, and become diluted within, the growing volume and streams of air they encounter. This mixing is not necessarily uniform and can be influenced by thermal layering and initial jetting of exhalations.
2. **Progressive loss of viral viability and infectiousness** over time is influenced by environmental factors such as temperature, humidity, and ultraviolet radiation (e.g., sunlight).

Transmission of SARS-CoV-2 from inhalation of virus in the air farther than six feet from an infectious source can occur.[44]

The CDC further reports that the Delta variant causes more infections and spreads faster than earlier forms of the virus that causes Covid-19. It might cause more severe illness than previous strains in unvaccinated people.[45]

Covid-19 vaccines are effective at helping protect against severe disease and death from variants of the virus that causes Covid-19 currently circulating, including the Delta variant. Infections happen in only a small proportion of people who are fully vaccinated, even with the Delta variant.

When these infections occur among vaccinated people, they tend to be mild. People who are fully vaccinated and become infected with the Delta variant might be able to spread the virus to others.

Those with weakened immune systems, including people who take immunosuppressive medications, may not be protected even if fully vaccinated.[46]

Chapter Six
What Was and Wasn't Done

KEY FACTS

- Emphasis on avoiding exposure, limiting spread, developing a vaccine
- Prevention recommendations include physical distancing, masks, ventilation
- Precautions largely overlooked how to boost the body's natural defenses

As the Covid-19 pandemic spread across the globe, the U.S. government initiated Operation Warp Speed, a $10 billion public-private partnership to develop and distribute vaccines, therapeutics and diagnostics.[47]

The U.S. Food and Drug Administration (FDA) reports that several vaccines have been developed and have Emergency Use Authorization (EUA) to ensure wide availability and deployment as countermeasures against the Covid-19 pandemic.

According to the FDA, under such emergency measures, it has the authority to use approved or unapproved medical products to diagnose, treat, or prevent serious or life-threatening diseases or conditions when certain criteria are met.

Manufacturers can submit a EUA request to the FDA which may or may not be approved considering all available scientific evidence and are expected to continue medical trials during the review process.[48] A couple of these vaccines have since received full FDA approval.[49]

Prevention recommendations from the CDC focused on physical means to reduce or stop transmission, with rarely any mention of increasing the body's ability to fight the virus and reduce the severity of symptoms or incidence of mortality.

Constant updates of new cases and deaths created a sense of panic. An unseen enemy seemed to be lurking around every corner, and every person was a possible source of infection.

The authorities across the world used essentially the same game plan to forestall the spread of the illness. Lockdowns, physical distancing, and masking were the chosen tools, but this caused a lot of economic distress. Governments in North America and elsewhere intervened to provide additional income supports to their citizens.

The CDC says the infectious dose of SARS-CoV-2 needed to transmit infection has not been established. Current evidence strongly suggests transmission from contaminated surfaces does not contribute substantially to new infections.

Although animal studies and epidemiologic investigations (in addition to those described above) indicate that inhalation of virus can cause infection, the relative contributions of inhalation of virus and deposition of the virus on mucous membranes remain unquantified and will be difficult to establish.

Despite these knowledge gaps, the available evidence continues to demonstrate that existing recommendations to prevent SARS-CoV-2 transmission remain effective.

These include physical distancing, community use of well-fitting masks (e.g., barrier face coverings, procedure/surgical masks), adequate ventilation, and avoidance of crowded indoor spaces. These methods will reduce transmission both from inhalation of the virus and deposition of the virus on exposed mucous membranes.

Transmission through soiled hands and surfaces can be prevented by practicing good hand hygiene and by environmental cleaning.[50]

The Mayo Clinic recommended the following precautions for avoiding exposure to Covid-19: [51]

- Avoid close contact (within about 6 feet, or 2 meters) with anyone who is sick or has symptoms.
- Keep distance between yourself and others (within about 6 feet, or 2 meters). This is especially important if you have a higher risk of serious illness. Keep in mind some people may have COVID-19 and spread it to others, even if they don't have symptoms or don't know they have COVID-19.
- Avoid crowds and indoor places that have poor ventilation.
- Wash your hands often with soap and water for at least 20 seconds or use an alcohol-based hand sanitizer that contains at least 60% alcohol.
- Wear a face mask in indoor public spaces and outdoors where there is a high risk of COVID-19 transmission, such as at a crowded event or large gathering. Further mask guidance differs depending on whether you are fully vaccinated or unvaccinated. Surgical masks may be used if available. N95 respirators should be reserved for health care providers.

- Cover your mouth and nose with your elbow or a tissue when you cough or sneeze. Throw away the used tissue. Wash your hands right away.
- Avoid touching your eyes, nose, and mouth.
- Avoid sharing dishes, glasses, towels, bedding, and other household items if you're sick.
- Clean and disinfect high-touch surfaces, such as doorknobs, light switches, electronics, and counters, daily.
- Stay home from work, school, and public areas if you're sick unless you're going to get medical care. Avoid public transportation, taxis and ridesharing if you're sick.
- If you have a chronic medical condition and may have a higher risk of serious illness, check with your doctor about other ways to protect yourself.

The CDC recommends against the use of any pre-exposure drugs except for participants in a clinical trial. It also admits there are no known agents to prevent infection despite various claims to the contrary.[52]

The WHO says that certain nutrients such as vitamins D, C and zinc are important for a healthy immune system, but it warns against any claims that vitamin or mineral supplements can cure a Covid-19 infection.[53]

For therapeutic management of Covid-19 in non-hospitalized situations, the CDC recommends over-the-counter antipyretics [acetaminophen, ibuprofen], analgesics [painkillers], or antitussives for fever, headache, myalgias, and cough [cough suppressants or expectorants].

Patients with dyspnea [shortness of breath] may benefit from resting in the prone [face down] position rather than the supine [face up] position. Health care providers should consider educating patients about breathing exercises, as severe breathlessness may cause anxiety.

Patients should be advised to drink fluids regularly to avoid dehydration. Rest is recommended as needed during the acute phase of Covid-19, and ambulation and other forms of activity should be increased according to the patient's tolerance.

Patients should be educated about the variability in time to symptom resolution and complete recovery.[54]

A study published in January 2021 in the American Journal of Respiratory and Critical Care Medicine observed that none of the major health authorities offered substantive recommendations about enhancing the body's immune system in the early treatment of Covid-19 and no treatment guidelines for those who exhibited symptoms beyond the general advice to stay home, rest, and go to a hospital if symptoms progressed.[55]

Chapter Seven
What Could Be Done

KEY FACTS

- More recommendations to boost the natural immune system
- More holistic understanding of immunity that includes both germ and terrain theory
- Germ theory sees external germs, viruses, and pathogens as the cause of disease
- Terrain theory sees the health of the human body playing a major role in mitigating infection
- More discussion on natural immunity that provides lasting immunity

There is an underreporting of the role the body's immune system plays in developing immunity to viruses.

Dr. Jennifer Nuzzo, an epidemiologist at the Johns Hopkins Center for Health Security, clarified the role of vaccines. "They don't prevent infections. They train your immune system to respond quickly to infections and hopefully limit the number of cells that get infected. They work to limit infections to prevent severe disease, hopefully, to keep people out of the hospital." [56]

Science magazine says that natural immunity provides the best and longest-lasting protection against SARS-CoV-2, even against the Delta variant. While the body's immune system is effective at developing antibodies in mild cases, the magazine emphasized that Covid-19 vaccines remain highly protective against serious illness or death. [57]

A study published by the Washington University School of Medicine similarly concluded that mild Covid-19 infections produced lasting antibodies.[58]

There are two main approaches to the study of disease transmission that help to explain why, when people are exposed to the same virus, some become very sick while others have no symptoms. Germ theory focuses on how external pathogens invade the body and cause disease. The theory was first devised by Louis Pasteur and now constitutes the foundations of Western medicine with an emphasis on developing antimicrobial drugs, vaccinations, and disinfectants to kill germs that might otherwise attack the body and transmit disease.[59]

Terrain theory, on the other hand, considers how disease fails to thrive in healthy bodies and tries to explain how a person's existing health status explains differences in how that person contracts and transmits the disease. Essentially, an unhealthy person is more susceptible to disease by providing germs with a better environment in which to thrive. When the body is in a homeostatic state of balance and health, its natural immune defenses do a better job of fighting off disease.[60]

Though not mutually exclusive approaches, in the context of the Covid-19 pandemic, there is an unbalanced emphasis on germ theory solutions that largely overlook the role that the body's natural defenses play in helping to fight disease.

A study published by the British Industrial Biological Research Association (BIBRA) found global responses to the Covid-19 pandemic focused on the virus itself but overlooked the contributing toxicological effects of populations with poor immune systems. The study observed that one of the major underlying causes of the pandemic include the fact that many people are vulnerable to the virus due to poor health. Confirmation of this can be drawn from the fact that most deaths attributed to Covid-19 included comorbidities such as hypertension, diabetes, cardiovascular disease, chronic respiratory disease, immune-compromised status, cancer, and obesity. Nearly 95% of Covid-19 deaths listed one or more comorbidities.[61]

According to the study, factors that impair the immune system include:

- Lifestyle: lack of exercise, smoking, excessive alcohol consumption, a poor diet of processed foods, sugar, and refined grains, and sleep deprivation
- Pharmaceutical drugs: More than half of adults 65 and older (54%) report taking four or more prescription drugs
- Biotoxins like mold, viruses, and bacteria
- Environmental exposures to things like endocrine disruptors, radiation and Wi-Fi, heavy metals, PFAS, fine particulate matter and many others
- Psychosocial factors like depression and stress.

The BIBRA study went on to observe that a variety of factors determine susceptibility to a disease beyond lifestyle and environmental toxins. Yet, millions of Americans can be considered nutrient deficient, and official responses to the pandemic largely do not include information about how to fight the virus with healthier immune systems. The study concluded that both tactical (immediate) and strategic (long-term) responses to the current pandemic are required.[62]

The National Institutes of Health reports that 95% of people who recovered from Covid-19 had developed effective antibodies to the virus, which helped support the science behind vaccines that hope to induce similar "immune memories" in the body.[63]

Dr. Mark Hyman, M.D., Head of Strategy and Innovation of the Cleveland Clinic Center for Functional Medicine and Board President for Clinical Affairs for The Institute for Functional Medicine, says the focus on assigning standardized treatments to sufferers should come second to a proactive focus on building natural immunity. Hyman points to the number of deaths with comorbidities, noting that given the prevalence of chronic disease and obesity in the American population, there are millions of people likely to develop a heightened inflammatory response to the virus.[64]

Dr. William Li, M.D., a physician, scientist, and founder of the Angiogenesis Foundation, similarly highlights the body's potential for natural immunity. He argues that harnessing the body's power to heal itself helps protect it against pathogens that cause infection and disease. He notes the body has three lines of defense: 1) innate, which includes barriers such as the skin, mucous, nails, etc., 2) cellular defenses, such as when white blood cells kill foreign substances, and 3) adaptive immunity, B lymphocytes that create antibodies to neutralize toxins and other invaders and hold the memory of these invasions to help create immunity to future invasions. He says that boosting our innate or adaptive immunity is key to protecting against disease.[65]

A study published by the T. Collin Campbell Center for Nutrition Studies similarly emphasizes the power of natural immunity and the body's ability to combat bacteria, viruses, parasites, toxins, chemicals, pollutants, and other stressors.[66]

Chapter Eight
Vitamin D and the Immune System

KEY FACTS

- Vitamin D plays a vital role in boosting the immune system
- A healthy immune system is critical to fighting infectious diseases
- Vitamin D deficiency increases susceptibility to infection

There is compelling evidence to suggest that vitamin D is a key part of maintaining a healthy immune system. In the context of the Covid-19 pandemic, vitamin D thus plays an important role in helping prevent the spread of infectious diseases.

In 2012, the Proceedings of the Nutrition Society observed that the effects of vitamin D on the immune system have been recognized for at least twenty-five years but only recently have become widely understood in terms of its effects on normal human physiology.

This change in perspective can be seen as owing to a growing volume of literature that connects vitamin insufficiency with immune disorders as well as increasing evidence of the link between vitamin D and a well-functioning immune system.[67]

According to a 2020 study published in Nutrients, a peer-reviewed scientific journal, vitamin D plays an important role in the immune system. When immune cells are exposed to vitamin D in scientific tests, there is a measurable physiological reaction.

In a controlled study of vitamin D deficiency in animals and humans, the immune system was impaired by the lack of vitamin D in the body. Regular supplementation of vitamin D on a daily or weekly dose can enhance the immune system and help to avoid vitamin D deficiency that can decrease susceptibility to autoimmune disease.[68]

A 2015 study published in the Journal of Investigative Medicine concluded that immune cells (B cells, T cells, antigen-presenting cells) are capable of synthesizing vitamin D in the body and acting upon innate and adaptive immune responses.

Vitamin D deficiency is therefore associated with autoimmune diseases and increased susceptibility to infection.[69]

These conclusions were shared by another study published in the journal Clinical Calcium.[70]

In Maturitas, a peer-reviewed medical journal, a recent study investigated the role of vitamin D supplementation in the context of Covid-19. The study concluded that adequate vitamins and minerals were essential to ensure proper immune function.

Dietary sources of vitamins D, C, E, zinc, and omega-3 fatty acids are important, but supplementation with higher doses during a Covid-19 infection have been shown to have positive outcomes.

These findings are particularly relevant to elderly and immunocompromised patients where dietary intake may not be sufficient to improve disease outcomes and elevated intake of key vitamins and minerals may be recommended.[71]

Chapter Nine
Covid Long-Haulers Share Their Roads to Recovery

Written by Adriana Velez
Reviewed by Jessica Rodriguez CNP

Most people recover from COVID-19 within two weeks. Not these survivors.

At the beginning of 2021, the United States finds itself at an inflection point of the COVID-19 pandemic. Over 400,000 people have died. The vaccine is rolling out, if in an uncoordinated manner. Researchers say we have reached the peak of the surge. But for many survivors, the battle is far from over.

Coronavirus long-haulers experience a range of symptoms, most commonly fatigue, brain fog, shortness of breath, joint pain, and chest pain.

Most people recover from COVID-19 within two weeks. Yet a smaller cohort of survivors, about 10 percent according to recent estimates, experience long-term health issues for four weeks or longer. These Coronavirus long-haulers experience a range of symptoms, most commonly fatigue (especially following bouts of physical activity), brain fog, shortness of breath, joint pain, and chest pain.

Other reported symptoms include everything from depression to hair loss to renal disease to the onset of type 2 diabetes.

As you might imagine, long-term COVID-19 is incredibly disruptive to a person's life. Months after their initial recovery from the Coronavirus, many long-haulers still require reduced work schedules, or are no longer working.

To get a clearer picture of what life is like for Coronavirus long-haulers on a personal level, we spoke with two survivors with very different stories.

Heather-Elizabeth Brown

Nine months after falling ill with COVID-19, Heather-Elizabeth Brown, a 36-year-old corporate trainer in Detroit, Michigan is still recovering.

Like many other people who were infected early in the pandemic, she was caught in the tangle of overwhelmed hospitals, inaccurate testing, and inexperience treating a new and terrifying virus.

In early April, Brown came down with a fever and was feeling fatigued. As a volunteer chaplain for the police who was fortunate enough to qualify as a first responder, she was able to get tested for the Coronavirus.

It came back negative. She was relieved, at first. But her symptoms worsened over the next four or five days, so she got another test. Again, it came back negative.

"I knew I was sick, and it wasn't just the flu. I didn't understand why I was getting these negative test results."

"At that point, I knew that I was sick, and it wasn't just the flu. I didn't understand why I was getting these negative test results," Brown says.

A telehealth nurse practitioner told her she had all the symptoms of COVID-19, but that some of the tests had up to a 33 percent rate of false results.

Brown was advised to continue self isolating. Her fever rose, and she started having gastrointestinal issues.

As her symptoms became even more severe, Brown went to the emergency room, or to be more accurate, she arrived at the drive-through screening. That's how things were in Detroit, New York, and other cities around the country by mid-April.

Hospitals were beyond capacity and emergency rooms did not have the space to keep potentially infected patients far enough apart.

Brown was told that as ill as she was, she did not meet the criteria to be admitted, and was sent home. She returned to the emergency room a second time and could not get a test but was given a positive diagnosis based on her symptoms in the absence of an available test.

As she wasn't in obvious respiratory distress and her oxygen levels weren't dangerously low, doctors prescribed hydroxychloroquine and told her to get a pulse oximeter. She was sent home yet again.

"I remember being at home that evening and telling my mom that I felt like if I went to sleep, I wouldn't wake up."

"I remember being at home that evening and telling my mom that I felt like if I went to sleep, I wouldn't wake up," Brown recalls. Her fever spiked to 103, she was having trouble breathing, and now her oxygen levels had dipped dangerously low. It hurt to breathe.

A third time she went to the emergency room. A third time she took a COVID test. Finally, it came out positive. A chest x-ray revealed she already had advanced COVID-induced pneumonia and she was told that she finally was sick enough to be admitted to the hospital to receive treatment.

Black, Latinx, and Indigenous people are four times as likely to be hospitalized from COVID-19, according to the CDC

At this point in the story, it's hard not to speculate how things might have been different if Brown had received the kind of care she needed at the earliest signs of symptoms. She is Black, which puts her at an elevated risk for becoming infected with COVID-19 in the first place, suffering more complications, and dying.

Black, Latinx, and Indigenous people are four times as likely to be hospitalized from the virus, according to the CDC. On social media, stories of inadequate care for BIPOC have been circulating, such as a video from Indianapolis doctor Susan Moore, who later died.

Another woman, whose entire family was infected, spoke out recently via Twitter that her mother was told by her white doctor not to go to the hospital unless her or her children's lips turned blue. "She's Black. Her lips will not turn blue," @DaniAtomicus tweeted.

Doctors put Brown into a medically-induced coma and on a ventilator. She would stay on that ventilator, in that coma, for 31 days, from April 18th to May 19th.

"It was a completely surreal experience," Brown says. Her brain was still active, and she had vivid dreams. Waking was also surreal. "I remember opening my eyes and people coaching me to breathe," she says. The first few days were a confusing, disorienting blur.

"Everything had to be explained to me, because I had been out for so long. Nothing made sense. When they were telling me what day it was, and they turned on the TV, I was like, what's going on?"

Brown remained in the ICU for another week and was released from the hospital on June 1st. But she has had to return numerous times. She was treated for blood clots in her leg, and complications from those clots.

During her month in the coma, she suffered a stroke while on the ventilator, lost the ability to walk, and the left side of her body became weak.

Between that and the painful blood clots, she had to re-learn how to walk through inpatient rehab, working her way out of a wheelchair into a walker until she would walk unassisted.

"I still had the expectation that my body was going to bounce back, especially when it came to the physical therapy part and walking again."

Doctors prepared Brown for a long recovery. There is no standard timeline, of course, but she was told to expect at least three days of recovery for every one day her body was inactive.

"I didn't have any grandiose dreams of running a marathon after I got off the ventilator," Brown says. But she was 35 when she fell ill, and in that younger demographic of people who tend to recover faster than older survivors

"I still had the expectation that my body was going to bounce back, especially when it came to the physical therapy part and walking again," Brown says. She was frustrated with how long it took her to stand and walk. Doctors told her it could be six to nine months.

"Some of us have that Superman complex, like they said it'll be this long for me, but I can do it a little bit faster. That hasn't happened," she says.

Brown is aware of the possibility of medical bias, but she doesn't like to look back and wonder, "What if?" First of all, it makes her sad.

Secondly, she points out that she benefited from her education, having health insurance, and her first responder status.

She emphasizes that she knows firsthand how overwhelmed hospitals were at that time. "I think everyone was trying their very, very best," she says. "I truly believe that."

Several months later Brown is still dealing with a chronic lung condition that may stay with her for the rest of her life. She's still in pulmonary rehab, and she struggles with fatigue and brain fog. In November she was diagnosed with type 2 diabetes.

This came as a surprise, especially since she had not been prediabetic before COVID-19.

In addition to her recovery, Brown now has to learn how to manage diabetes, which for her includes injecting insulin multiple times a day.

"On top of the adjustment of having to deal with diabetes as a health concern, there's also the emotional and psychological part of giving myself injections because I absolutely hate needles."

She's hoping that her glucose levels will stabilize, she'll be able to drop insulin, and she's grateful for the use of a continuous glucose monitor.

Even Brown's eyesight has changed, probably because of the diabetes. Her eyeglass prescription has shifted by five points, the biggest shift her optometrist had ever seen. She was prescribed temporary contact lenses because her prescription changes every other week.

Another stressful aspect of long-haul COVID is how little we still know about it, and how dramatically it disrupts our sense of security

Another stressful aspect of long-haul COVID is how little we still know about it, and how dramatically it disrupts our sense of security. "This is something that's new and there's not a lot of information about what to do and how to do it," Brown says.

"Everyone's just kind of playing it by ear and learning as we go." Clear answers are hard to come by, and that's difficult to face if you've always expected that the medical world will be there to cure you, no matter what happens.

"We take for granted the idea that if something goes wrong, doctors will be able to fix us. We assume there will always be ample space in hospitals for our treatment. What we're seeing is that there are serious limits to how many people hospitals can treat at one time," she says.

Given all of this, it's a good thing Brown has a strong support network, starting with her family. Her parents, who are in their 70s, live in Mississippi, but her mother and an uncle came to Michigan to be with Brown while she was in the hospital.

They stayed with her for another three and a half months to help with her recovery. Brown also has a large "church family" from Citadel of Praise in Detroit who have brought her meals, made deliveries, and provided other kinds of everyday support.

Meanwhile, Brown's employer has also been a source of relief. She had just started working for Quicken Loans in March, on the job for all of three weeks before she fell ill.

"My company was really supportive," she says. They held her position for her and stayed in contact with her mother for updates.

When Brown wanted to start working again part time just to regain a sense of normalcy in her life, Quicken made accommodations for her, enabling her to work around her numerous doctors appointments.

Between physical and pulmonary therapy, blood tests, and other check-ins, Brown has four to five appointments a week. "We know you want to come back, and we'll figure out a way to make it work," her employers keep telling her.

Not feeling pressured to get back to full-time hours makes a huge difference in helping her recovery.

Brown's COVID-19 ordeal has forced her to acknowledge her fragility as a human being, and to confront her mortality "in a very real and tangible way." Faith plays a large role in dealing with the ups and downs of her now chronic illness.

"I've had to lean heavily on my faith to get me through some of some of the more challenging diagnoses and painful moments," she says.

Then there is the COVID-19 support group Brown found with Body Politic, a queer, feminist wellness collective.

"Before I found Body Politic, I was actually in a different community. It was a Facebook group for people with COVID. "I kind of felt a little out of place," she says diplomatically.

Other members were talking about having a slight fever and body aches, or cabin fever on day three of quarantine. "It felt weird. I'm supposed to be like, 'I just got out of 31-day coma'?"

When she came across an article about Body Politic, she felt like she'd finally found people with the same depth of experience she had. The group shares information about testing, recovery, news, and even the terms associated with COVID-19.

"It was really helpful, being able to read and realize that there was a larger community I could identify with. Just knowing that you're not the only one out there."

"Even in the midst of what happened, the fact is that I survived, and I now have the opportunity to have these conversations and to be an advocate for other COVID long-haulers."

Through all her ordeals, Brown now finds herself in a place of gratitude for her life, of grace and acceptance. She is also buoyed by a greater sense of purpose. "I am where I am.

Even in the midst of what happened, the fact is that I survived, and I now have the opportunity to have these conversations and to be an advocate for other COVID long-haulers," she says.

"I hope that people will continue to realize that this virus is real, that it's dangerous, and that they do what they need to do to protect not only themselves, but other people in our communities who are most vulnerable.

It's important to continue to adhere to the guidelines, even if it's a killjoy. We have to be community-minded. We have to realize that one person may get it and it may not affect them severely.

But if they transmit it to someone else, they may not be as lucky. They may not have the same presentation. That's what's most important, is not only protecting ourselves, but protecting everyone else."

Amanda Thebe

A "moderate" case of the Coronavirus that stretched on for 17 weeks

When Amanda Thebe, a 50-year-old fitness expert and menopause educator in Houston, Texas, developed itchy eyes and a sore throat towards the end of March, she thought she had allergies.

Antihistamines didn't help. She picked up a bad cough and started wheezing, and still she thought it might be allergies, maybe combined with a cold. Three weeks later, she was feeling worse and came down with a fever that wouldn't go away. When she started having trouble breathing, she went to a hospital for a COVID-19 test.

"I started going out for these little walks, but they were just so difficult. When I'd come home, I'd have to go back to bed for two or three days to recover."

The test confirmed that Thebe had the Coronavirus, but her case was relatively moderate at the time. She was able to convalesce at home without hospitalization. Three weeks later, she started "feeling human" again, except for a tenaciously severe fatigue she couldn't shake

"I started going out for these little walks, but they were just so difficult. When I'd come home, I'd have to go back to bed for two or three days to recover," she says.

At first Thebe thought she was pushing herself too hard, too soon. But as the weeks slipped by, and her fatigue persisted (especially after any physical activity, such as walking), and she knew this was no ordinary recovery.

It would be another 17 weeks from the time she emerged from the worst of the virus before she started feeling close to the way she had before.

"It was crazy," she recalls. "I just couldn't do everyday things. I couldn't walk up the stairs. I had terrible shortness of breath, chronic fatigue, the type of stuff you can't sleep off."

It reminded her of her battle with perimenopause (which she documented in her book, Menopocalypse), when she had severe and confusing symptoms. This time, she felt desperate and isolated.

Fortunately, Thebe's thoughtful primary physician saw similarities between her symptoms and those of post-viral syndrome, a disease that can follow a viral infection, and which causes chronic fatigue.

He told Thebe that it could take her four to six months before she turned a corner. He admitted doctors still had much to learn about this post-COVID-19 condition, but that he would try to do what he could to help her feel better.

Thebe went on a course of steroids and other medications to reduce inflammation. She started seeing a pulmonologist for her shortness of breath and chest pain.

Surprisingly, that doctor started treating her for acid reflux. Gastrointestinal problems like GERD (gastroesophageal acid reflux) are a less-known, but fairly common symptoms among COVID-19 patients.

As a former fitness trainer who loves lifting weights, swimming, and all manner of exercise, taking a break from physical activity was disappointing but necessary.

Thanks to her experience with perimenopause, Thebe already knew how to scale back to accommodate her energy levels.

Still, she admits feeling demoralized at times as she gradually began introducing movement back into her life.

"Even when it went on for months and months, I kept saying 'I'm sorry, I feel like a failure.'"

"At home, I didn't want to admit that I was sick, so I was trying to push through," Thebe says. "My family was amazing. They could clearly see that I still wasn't well."

Her husband and two teenage sons kept making her sit down and rest every time she attempted household tasks. "Even when it went on for months and months, I kept saying 'I'm sorry, I feel like a failure.'"

Thebe admits she was harder on herself than anyone else. She felt especially bad because she'd had such a difficult time with perimenopause years earlier, and now here she was, struggling with post-COVID fatigue as well.

She also felt guilty about contracting COVID-19 in the first place, as if she'd done something wrong, even though she'd been very careful about wearing a mask and social distancing.

It helped when one of Thebe's friends texted her, "You have to quit talking like this. There's so much we don't know about this disease, and you've been hit so hard. Please stop apologizing for it."

Fortunately, Thebe joined Survivor Corps, a support group founded by COVID long-hauler Diane Berrent. It was through this group that she found out how common gastrointestinal issues were, and how many other survivors have been left with seemingly permanent conditions.

Fortunately, CT scans show no permanent damage to Thebe's lungs and heart.

"But there are people with lung scarring, and they're simply not recovering," she says.

Thanks to the support of family, friends, and Survivor Corps, Thebe had the courage to start talking about her long recovery on her Instagram.

"It garnered so much attention because people were like, 'I've got it too, and I'm not recovering. Thank you, it's really helpful to know how you're doing.'"

Now, all these months later, Thebe is happy to report that she's feeling "super-fit and healthy" again. She does have some residual gastrointestinal issues, but they're manageable. She's aware that other long-haulers are still struggling and trying to solve the mysteries behind their protracted recovery.

"The way we talk about health sometimes, we add a kind of layer of morality on it, like if you're not healthy it's your fault. There's so much we still don't understand about this Coronavirus, and there are so many factors outside of our control."

That's why Thebe wants to give her fellow Coronavirus long-haulers a glimmer of hope that they can recover at least some of their energy and vitality. More than that, she thinks it's important that people not feel shame.

"The way we talk about health sometimes, we add a kind of layer of morality on it, like if you're not healthy, it's your fault," Thebe says. "There's so much we still don't understand about this virus, and there are so many factors outside of our control."

At first, Thebe wanted to know why her recovery was taking so long. She followed her natural curiosity, and started reading all of the research she could find. She tried alternative treatments. She wondered if there was some underlying cause.

Was it because she had an uncommon blood type? "I needed answers so that I could stop blaming myself," Thebe says. It was her primary care physician who finally told her, "We may never know why, and you need to accept that."

This acceptance of the unknown has been an important piece of Thebe's emotional recovery from long-haul COVID-19.

Another turning point for Thebe was finding a guide to managing post-viral fatigue from the National Health Service in the UK. As an athlete, Thebe's practice had always been to push her physical limits. But she learned that when it comes to long-haul COVID-19, this was the exact opposite of what she needed.

In this case, exercise was not necessarily her friend. The post-viral fatigue guide "spoke about fatigue, and it talked about working within an energy envelope," she says.

In other words, doing a little bit less than what you think you can (or should) do is the most helpful strategy. When Thebe wanted to take a walk, she would go out for only five minutes, even if she felt she could last for ten.

Thebe's practice became what she calls "fitness snacking," tiny bits of exercise that made her feel better, but that didn't push her energy levels at all. Working within that energy envelope was another pivotal moment for Thebe.

Along with a commitment to eating the most nutrient-dense food she could and staying hydrated, this approach helped her both physically and mentally. Even better, sharing her approach has helped other COVID long-haulers following Thebe's social media.

"It makes them feel like they're getting small wins as well," she says. "Overtime, those small wins can make a huge difference."

Last updated on 6/23/2021

Reprinted with permission from EndocrineWeb, a property of Remedy Health Media. www.EndocrineWeb.com

03

Treatments For Long Haul Covid

Chapter Ten
Choosing Your Own Path

There are a variety of treatments being advocated for relieving the symptoms of long haul Covid. Different groups and organizations, comprised of health professionals such as the CDC and the major medical centers and some formed by patients, offer their suggestions and remedies.

Many treatments recommended in online self-help groups have proven helpful to long haul Covid sufferers.

Unfortunately, there seems to be a bewildering number of approaches – some work for some, and many do not seem to provide the needed relief.

This part of the book will summarize a number of these treatments. I am not a health professional, and none of these treatments described is medical advice.

My sole aim is to inform you of these different treatments so you can inform yourself about the choices available and discuss them with your healthcare provider.

As you will see, there is not any consensus. On the contrary, some may oppose each other.

It thus falls to you to do your homework, to try to identify those treatments that might help alleviate your symptoms and find the health professionals who can help guide you along your chosen path.

In addition, of course, you must consider the potential toxicity of any treatment and minimize any adverse effects on your body.

You may find your current health provider is not in agreement with your choices. Then you will have a decision to make – either strike out on your own and find the help you want or stick with your current provider, which can be nerve-racking as there is no guarantee that the treatment you wish to pursue will work in your case.

It can sometimes take a brave act of courage to determine for yourself how best to treat your long haul Covid.

Too often, we have only listened to conventional medical authorities on how to treat chronic conditions. Unfortunately, traditional medicine has not proven to be very effective in treating chronic conditions.

It tends to focus on suppressing the symptoms rather than treating the root cause of the chronic disease.

With long haul Covid, we have a chronic disease that affects the whole body with over 200 symptoms. These can range through all the major organ systems – the lungs, heart, liver, skin and brain.

It has such a diversity of symptoms that one hardly knows where to start. Similarly, this roadmap offers an assortment of treatment options.

It will be up to you and your healthcare provider to find those that work best for you.

Chapter Eleven
CDC Guidance on Treating Long Haul Covid

KEY FACTS

- Health care providers and patients must work together to set goals and plans
- Mild illness can be treated with supportive care aimed at relieving symptoms
- Several agents are being investigated including Ivermectin, vitamin D and interferons
- Recommendations against the use of drugs unless as part of a clinical trial

The Centres for Disease Control and Prevention (CDC) offers guidelines regarding the treatment of long haul Covid, which they define as patients experiencing illness at least four weeks after acute infection of the Covid-19 virus. Primary care providers are the first line of defense and can often be relied upon to treat symptoms and establish a comprehensive management plan.

For most patients, the goal of medical management of post-Covid conditions is to optimize function and quality of life. Ideally, healthcare professionals, in consultation with the appropriate specialists, should develop a comprehensive management plan based on their patients' presenting symptoms, underlying medical and psychiatric conditions, personal and social situations, and their treatment goals.[72]

In evaluating and caring for patients with post-Covid 19 conditions the CDC offers the following guidance:[73]

- The term "Post-Covid Conditions" is an umbrella term for the wide range of physical and mental health consequences experienced by some patients that are present four or more weeks after SARS-CoV-2 infection, including by patients who had an initial mild or asymptomatic acute infection.
- Based on current information, many post-Covid conditions can be managed by primary care providers, with the incorporation of patient-centered approaches to optimize the quality of life and function in affected patients.
- Objective laboratory or imaging findings should not be used as the only measure or assessment of a patient's well-being; lack of laboratory or imaging abnormalities does not invalidate the existence, severity, or importance of a patient's symptoms or conditions.
- Healthcare professionals and patients are encouraged to set achievable goals through shared decision-making and to approach treatment by focusing on specific symptoms (e.g., headache) or conditions (e.g., dysautonomia); a comprehensive management plan focusing on improving physical, mental, and social wellbeing may be helpful for some patients.
- Understanding of post-Covid conditions remains incomplete and guidance for healthcare professionals will likely change over time as the evidence evolves.

Chapter Twelve
Towards A Multidisciplinary Approach

KEY FACTS

- Multidisciplinary teams are key as symptoms are not typically restricted to just one organ system
- The goal is to provide a central resource for patients with specialists from diverse clinical practices
- Patients are often dismissed from other clinics as having imagined their symptoms

Multidisciplinary clinics have been established in many major hospitals to support Covid-19 patients and help long haul Covid patients whose symptoms are diverse and often include more than one organ system. The Dana–Farber Cancer Institute says multidisciplinary teams often consist of specialists in respiratory, critical care, infectious diseases, psychiatry, and psychological services. These teams have been established at clinics such as Stanford Health Center, Mayo Clinic, Michigan Medicine, Johns Hopkins Medicine, Penn Medicine and UC Davis.[74]

An NBC News investigation of sixty-four post-Covid clinics in March 2021 found there was no standard of treatment for post-Covid-19 patients.

Some therapies included physical therapy while others focused on mindfulness with varying degrees of success since patient needs are so different.

In many cases, it's unclear which specialist a patient needs to address their symptoms given post-Covid is such a new disease, and the rise in the number of post-Covid patients will spur research into the syndrome.

NBC News found that clinicians often must rely on experience with other long-term illnesses, such as chronic fatigue, fibromyalgia, and post-intensive care syndrome given the number of Covid-19 patients that spend time in ICUs.

Many patients reported feeling abandoned when they were turned away from other clinics and healthcare providers unable or unwilling to help them.[75]

Post-Covid recovery programs aim to provide a central resource for patients that begin with a comprehensive assessment and care plan that involves referrals to various specialists.

Treatment plans often follow that of established programs for similar conditions, such as chronic obstructive pulmonary disease (COPD), heart issues, concussion, and transplant patients.

A typical team might include infectious disease specialists, pulmonary medicine doctors, primary care doctors, cardiologists, kidney specialists, physical and occupational therapists, radiologists, neurologists, therapists, social workers, and pharmacists.[76]

Chapter Thirteen
Treating Long Haul Covid as a Chronic Disease

KEY FACTS

- Long haul Covid patients must borrow from other treatment plans
- Experts in post-intensive care syndrome pivoting to help long haul Covid patients
- Underlying infections may predispose patients to develop more severe Covid-19

A complementary approach that is becoming more widespread is approaching long haul Covid as a chronic disease and examining which complementary methods that prove successful with other chronic illnesses might prove helpful here.

In April 2021, The Atlantic magazine reported that academic medical centers are leading the way in developing a treatment for long Covid patients. The medical establishment has a long track record of being slow to recognize chronic illnesses and develop appropriate treatments. Long haul Covid patients are just the latest among groups of chronic disease sufferers who have faced disbelief by many physicians.

Fortunately, many trails have already been blazed by these other chronic diseases, which has helped to develop the idea that the immune system's response to disease can cause damage to the body.

There is growing evidence that Covid-19 damages lungs, heart, and even the brain, esophagus and other organs, requiring doctors to adopt a new perspective of disease that takes a more individualized view of the treatment of long Covid as a chronic disease.[77]

There is some research by Thomas Lewis, Ph.D. a microbiologist, and Dr. Michael Carter, an integrative physician, that focuses on identifying underlying chronic infections that undermine overall health.

Lewis and Carter run a company, Health Revival Partners, that performs diagnostic testing to help patients diagnose various ailments by pinpointing certain biomarkers that determine where an individual falls on a continuum of health/disease.[78] healthrevivalpartners.com

They conclude that infectious pathogens can trigger chronic diseases that can predispose a person to develop more severe Covid-19 symptoms. Such pathogens include those that attack the respiratory system.

If a patient has elevated white blood cell markers, there is the likelihood of an infection, a correlation that connects antibody levels to the risk of chronic disease.[79]

Chapter Fourteen
Functional Medicine Approach to Restoring Health

KEY FACTS

- A patient-centered approach focusing on the root cause of disease
- Comprehensive individualized treatment plans seek to restore health
- Nutrition plays a key role in healing

The Institute for Functional Medicine describes the functional medicine approach as seeking to determine the root cause of illness to restore health.

Instead of focusing on symptoms, functional medicine tries to address the causes of illness in an individual by considering the patient's potential for resiliency against infectious diseases, such as Covid-19.

It is an individualized, patient-centered model focused on the underlying causes of disease to achieve optimal health by evaluating genetic, biochemical and lifestyle factors to develop personalized treatment plans. Built into the approach is intrinsic flexibility to diagnose complex diseases.[80]

The Cleveland Clinic Center for Functional Medicine was established in 2014 as the first of its kind in the U.S., offering innovative approaches to chronic disease management

A comprehensive assessment is made of a patient's nutrition, stress, toxins, allergens, genetics, and microbiome to design a healthy living plan that outlines nutritional, exercise, and sleep needs, mental and emotional triggers. Food and nutrition play an especially important role as the primary component in a healing plan that empowers patients to take control of their health.[81]

The Institute for Functional Medicine defers first to all official sources and their recommendations to decrease transmission of viruses.

Beyond that, the Institute recommends that the functional medicine approach may boost the overall immune system by optimizing Covid-19 patients' "modifiable lifestyle," which may include enhancing the body's ability to fight infection and mitigate the damage of other therapeutics.

The Institute says that nutraceutical and other botanical agents that enhance the immune system "could potentially inhibit SARS-CoV-2 replication," including curcumin, echinacea, elderberry, licorice, vitamins A, C and D, among several others.[82]

An article written by Mo Perry, an editor of Experience Life, a wellness website, shares several functional medicine recommendations for Covid-19 sufferers, emphasizing the complex ways in which the virus attacks the body that promote a more holistic response.

An anti-inflammatory "food-first" approach is key with a diet low in refined carbohydrates and rich in protein, fiber, healthy fats and micronutrients, including zinc and selenium.

Other antioxidants and anti-inflammatory agents include the amino acid N-Acetyl-L-Cysteine (NAC), a polyphenol called resveratrol found in berries, intermittent fasting, probiotics, melatonin, a flavonoid called quercetin found in some fruits and vegetables, vitamin D, and other herbs and supplements.

Such strategies for treating long Covid are a starting point, Perry stresses, with each patient requiring a unique protocol developed by a practitioner based on the patient's environment, lifestyle, triggers, and history.[83]

Chapter Fifteen
Innovative Medical Protocols and Treatments

KEY FACTS

- *I-RECOVER FLCCC Management Protocol for Long Haul Covid Syndrome*
- *IncellDx SUSHI diagnostic tool*
- *Chronic Covid Diagnosis and Treatment Center*
- *Covid-19 vaccine for unvaccinated long Covid sufferers*
- *Ozone*
- *Naltrexone*

Several medical doctors have been developing innovative ways to help their patients overcome the debilitating effects of long haul Covid.

These doctors are on the front lines working with patients and have been developing some particularly innovative and non-conventional medical treatments, which have shown great success.

Their protocols are helping long haulers to recover.

In February 2021, a UK article in the Lancet Respiratory Medicine, a peer-reviewed journal for medicine and public policy, concluded that while many reports are describing long haul Covid "studies evaluating treatment options are glaringly sparse.[84]

The Front Line Covid-19 Critical Care Alliance (FLCCC) is a non-profit organization established in March 2020 by leading critical care specialists to develop effective treatment protocols to prevent the transmission of Covid-19 and improve outcomes for ill patients.[85]

Among FLCCC's highly respected members are Dr. Paul E. Marik, Professor of Medicine and Chief of the Division of Pulmonary and Critical Care Medicine at Eastern Virginia Medical School and a leading expert in the management of sepsis.

Dr. Marik is a prolific researcher and one of the most published and cited critical care physicians in the world with over 500 peer-reviewed articles, 80 book chapters and four critical care books. He is cited over 43,000 times.

Dr. Joseph Varon is Editor-in-Chief for Critical Care and Shock and Current Respiratory Medicine Reviews and is considered one of the top physicians in the United States, known for his contributions to the field of cardiopulmonary resuscitation and therapeutic hypothermia.

He has contributed to more than 830 peer-reviewed articles, 10 textbooks, and 15 book chapters in the medical literature.

Dr. Varon founded the Medical Prevention and Research Institute in Houston and was a co-developer of the MATH+ protocol to care for patients.

Dr. G. Umberton Meduri is one of the leading authorities on non-invasive ventilation for acute respiratory failure. He has over 120 peer-reviewed publications and has been cited 25,000 times.

These are just a few of the many leading FLCCC doctors whose published and front-line work is setting standards in the field of critical care.[86]

The lack of treatment recommendations for long haul Covid patients that incorporated empirical observations across the globe led the FLCCC to develop the I-RECOVER care management protocol.

Like other FLCCC protocols, I-RECOVER is a consensus-based guideline that evolves as clinical and scientific data emerges to provide direction to critical care doctors caring for patients with long haul Covid.

This approach also ensures frontline doctors have access to the most up-to-date guidance on caring for such patients.[87]

To learn more about the specific I RECOVER protocol visit this website: covid19criticalcare.com

Another innovator in the field of treatment for long haul Covid is Dr. Bruce Patterson. Former Medical Director of Diagnostic Virology at Standford University Hospitals and Clinics and specialist in viral pathogenesis, Dr. Patterson founded IncellDx, a medical diagnostic company that uses a specialized method called Simultaneous Ultrasensitive Signal-amplified Hybridization In Situ (SUSHI) to measure cell types in help with diagnosis and disease localization.[88]

The innovative approach analyzes the immune system to develop a profile of any abnormalities or impairments and decide what medications may work best, including recommendations for FDA approved drugs.[89]

Dr. Patterson has developed a Chronic Covid Diagnosis and Treatment Center in partnership with various research facilities, clinics and laboratories to provide long haul Covid patients with medical consultation and counseling to predict, diagnose and optimizing treatment.

Through ongoing research prevents any conclusive evidence, Dr. Patterson believes the cause of long haul Covid is due to "viral persistence, inactivated viral fragments, or reactivation of a latent virus."

Pro-inflammatory cytokines, immunoregulatory proteins made by immune cells that communicate and coordinate immune responses, are seen as the likely culprit behind chronic Covid-19 since elevated cytokines can contribute to hyperinflammation.

IncellDx's diagnostic tool is used to comprehensively evaluate cytokines to determine how the viral pathogens impair the immune system in patients.[90]

In a July 2021 interview with ETNT Health, a wellness website, Dr. Patterson explained that early in the pandemic, it became clear that Covid-19 patients discharged from the hospital continued to have symptoms three and four months following infection.

His team developed a machine learning AI computer program to compare the immune profiles of acute Covid-19 patients with long haulers, which led to the discovery of immunologic abnormalities in long haul Covid sufferers.

Vascular inflammation in long haulers appeared to be the biggest difference, inflicting damage in the lungs, chest, heart, and other organs. This led to the development of diagnostic panels specifically for Covid-19 and long Covid that generate a severity index and precision prescription of existing medications that can help in recovery.[91]

People seeking Dr. Patterson's long Covid diagnostic are directed to covidlonghaulers.com where they can register to have their blood sent for testing. A follow-up telemedicine appointment is made with one of his team's physicians to discuss the results, make recommendations and liaise with primary care physicians.[92]

Further discussion of Dr. Patterson's diagnostic protocols can be found on; youtube.com/watch?v=XWrCE3Ufi2c youtube.com/watch?v=9HSKceCt8tQ

In September 2021, a team at the University of Arkansas Medical Sciences published a study in PLOS ONE, a peer-reviewed scientific journal, investigating the role of an antibody that shows up in long Covid patients that disrupts the ACE2 enzyme which regulates the immune system.

By interfering with the proper functioning of the enzyme, this antibody is thought to be a major reason many Covid-19 patients develop lingering or new symptoms following infection.

The discovery promises to assist in further research to develop treatment models and drugs to help patients recover from symptoms.[93]

There is also growing evidence that the Covid-19 vaccine itself can help unvaccinated long Covid patients recover from symptoms, as reported in one WebMD article citing evidence from various public polls and surveys.

According to one such poll among 625 members of the SurvivorCorps long Covid patient advocacy group, approximately 40% saw an improvement of their symptoms following vaccination. Other doctors, such as Daniel Griffin, MD and Donna Farber, PhD at Columbia University indicate many people infected with Covid-19 felt better one- or two weeks following vaccination.

The inconclusive hypothesis among researchers is that the vaccination stimulates an immune response that helps to alleviate long Covid symptoms, though more studies are needed to confirm this.[94]

Since increasing numbers of studies see long Covid as a chronic inflammatory condition, ozone treatments may hold promise for helping relieve symptoms for long haul Covid sufferers.

According to a 2021 study published in the International Journal of Molecular Sciences, low-dose ozone has been found to help reduce symptoms associated with chronic inflammatory diseases. The treatment, either topical or systemic, works by stimulating various regulatory, signalling and antioxidizing responses within the body to help reduce inflammation.[95]

Two earlier studies from 2020 found that ozone therapy could be useful in combating coronaviruses, particularly in patients experiencing severe respiratory failure and may alleviate the need for invasive ventilation procedures.[96]

A 2014 study published in Clinical Rheumatology, a peer-reviewed medical journal on rheumatology, demonstrated that low-dose naltrexone, typically used to treat addiction by blocking certain opioid receptors, may be used as an anti-inflammatory agent in the central nervous system.

The study admits there is little research to support conclusive recommendations, but growing evidence of naltrexone treatments in patients with fibromyalgia, Crohn's disease, multiple sclerosis, and complex regional pain syndrome, suggests it may be a promising treatment approach for other chronic inflammatory diseases.[97]

There are ongoing pilot studies to investigate the treatment of naltrexone in patients with the post-Covid-19 syndrome.[98]

Chapter Sixteen
Complementary Treatments

KEY FACTS

- *Homeopathy*
- *Acupuncture*
- *Integrative medicine*

Long haulers are using several complementary treatments to mitigate the symptoms of long haul Covid.

These modalities lie outside the mainstream of conventional medicine, but there is evidence that they may offer some relief to the many long-haul symptoms.

Readers are responsible for their own choices in finding a healthcare practitioner willing to work with them to implement such complementary therapies.

Homeopathic medicine relies on the philosophy that the body is capable of healing itself. Dr. Vikas Sharma, MD, a homeopathy specialist, suggests homeopathy can be used to manage the symptoms of the post-Covid syndrome.

Homeopathic medicines are already used to treat many of these symptoms, including chronic fatigue, nausea, sleeplessness, muscle and joint pain, anxiety, brain fog and dizziness.

The selection and dosage of any such medicines should be done in consultation with a homeopathic physician.[99]

Acupuncture may also help relieve symptoms associated with long haul Covid. According to the Mayo Clinic, the practice of acupuncture involves inserting long metallic needles through the skin at various strategic points in the body to stimulate specific nerves, muscles and connective tissues that may help to relieve pain and promote overall wellness.[100]

A September 2021 study published in Briefings in Bioinformatics, a peer-reviewed scientific journal, revealed that acupuncture treatment for Covid-19 patients was associated with reduction of inflammation, improved immunity and nervous system function, with additional benefits for patients with certain comorbidities such as cancer, cardiovascular disease and obesity.[101]

The Harvard Gazette reported in 2020 that neuroscientists at Harvard Medical School used acupuncture to treat systemic inflammation in mice, successfully activating signaling pathways that triggered pro- and anti-inflammatory response.[102]

More information about acupuncture therapy can be found below;

ncbi.nlm.nih.gov/books/NBK532287

Integrative Medicine is a form of medical therapy that combines various complementary medicine treatments with conventional medical practice.

To learn more, readers are encouraged to review the 2020 article published in the Journal of Science and Healing, "Integrative medicine considerations for convalescence from mild-to-moderate COVID-19 disease," by Alschuler et al., available below;

sciencedirect.com/science/article/pii/S1550830720304171

The article concludes that integrative medicine can support convalescence from Covid-19 infection and outlines various treatments, including dietary supplements, osteopathic manipulation, qigong and other breathing exercises, pulmonary rehabilitation, stress management practices, aromatherapy, and sleep therapy.[103]

Chapter Seventeen
Canceling the Spike Protein
Striking Visual Evidence
Editorial by Thomas E. Levy, MD, JD

OMNS (Oct. 18, 2021) No issue in the history of medicine has been as strident and polarized as that of the risk/benefit profiles of the various COVID vaccines being administered around the world.

This article does not seek to clarify this issue to the satisfaction of either the pro-vaccine or the anti-vaccine advocates.

However, all parties should realize that *some* toxicity does result in *some* vaccinated individuals some of the time, and that such toxicity can *sometimes* be unequivocally attributed to the preceding administration of the vaccine.

Whether this toxicity occurs often enough and with great enough severity in vaccinated persons to be of greater concern than dealing with the contraction and evolution of COVID infections remains the question for many people.

Practically speaking, it does not matter whether an adverse event that occurs after a vaccination gets "blamed" on the vaccination. Such a matter may never get resolved.

The issue of greatest concern is whether that adverse event can be clinically resolved if not effectively prevented, and whether any long-term damage to the body can be prevented once an adverse event is recognized.

The remainder of this article will address the etiologies of such damage along with measures that can mitigate or even resolve such damage.

Toxins and Oxidative Stress

All toxins ultimately inflict their damage by directly oxidizing biomolecules, or by indirectly resulting in the oxidation of those biomolecules (proteins, sugars, fats, enzymes, etc.).

When biomolecules becomes oxidized (lose electrons) they can no longer perform their normal chemical or metabolic functions. No toxin can cause any clinical toxicity unless biomolecules end up becoming oxidized.

The unique array of biomolecules that become oxidized determines the nature of the clinical condition resulting from a given toxin exposure.

There is no "disease" present in a cell involved in a given medical condition beyond the distribution and degree of biomolecules that are oxidized.

Rather than "causing" disease, the state of oxidation in a grouping of biomolecules **IS** the disease.

When antioxidants can donate electrons back to oxidized biomolecules (reduction), the normal function of these biomolecules is restored (Levy, 2019).

This is the reason why sufficient antioxidant therapy, such as can be achieved by highly-dosed intravenous vitamin C, has proven to be so profoundly effective in blocking and even reversing the negative clinical impact of any toxin or poison.

There exists no toxin against which vitamin C has been tested that has not been effectively neutralized (Levy, 2002).

There is no better way to save a patient clinically poisoned by any agent than by immediately administering a sizeable intravenous infusion of sodium ascorbate.

The addition of magnesium chloride to the infusion is also important to protect against sudden life-threatening arrhythmias that can occur before a sufficient number of the newly-oxidized biomolecules can be reduced and any remaining toxin is neutralized and excreted.

Abnormal Blood Clotting

Both the COVID vaccine and the COVID infection have been documented to provoke increased blood clotting [thrombosis] (Biswas et al., 2021; Lundstrom et al., 2021).

Viral infections in general have been found to cause coagulopathies resulting in abnormal blood clotting (Subramaniam and Scharrer, 2018).

Critically ill COVID ICU patients demonstrated elevated D-dimer levels roughly 60% of the time (Iba et al., 2020).

An elevated D-dimer test result is almost an absolute confirmation of abnormal blood clotting taking place somewhere in the body.

Such clots can be microscopic, at the capillary level, or much larger, even involving the thrombosis of large blood vessels.

Higher D-dimer levels that persist in COVID patients appear to directly correlate with significantly increased morbidity and mortality (Naymagon et al., 2020; Paliogiannis et al., 2020; Rostami and Mansouritorghabeh, 2020).

Platelets, the elements of the blood that can get sticky and both initiate and help grow the size of blood clots, will generally demonstrate declining levels in the blood at the same time D-dimer levels are increasing, since their stores are being actively depleted.

A post-vaccination syndrome known as vaccine-induced prothrombotic immune thrombocytopenia (VIPIT) with these very findings has been described (Favaloro, 2021; Iba et al., 2021; Scully et al., 2021; Thaler et al., 2021).

Vaccinations have also been documented to cause bleeding syndromes due to autoimmune reactions resulting in low platelet levels (Perricone et al., 2014).

This can create some confusion clinically, as chronically low platelet levels by themselves can promote clinical syndromes of increased bleeding rather than increased blood clotting

As such, some primary low platelet disorders require pro-coagulation measures to stop bleeding, while other conditions featuring primary increased thrombosis with the secondary rapid consumption of platelet stores end up needing anticoagulation measures to stop that continued consumption of platelets (Perry et al., 2021).

Significant thrombosis post-vaccination in the absence of an elevated D-dimer level or low platelet count has also been described (Carli et al., 2021).

In platelets taken from COVID patients, platelet stickiness predisposing to thrombosis has been shown to result from spike protein binding to ACE2 receptors on the platelets (Zhang et al., 2021).

Of note, a D-dimer test that is elevated due to increased blood clotting will _**usually only stay elevated for a few days**_ after the underlying pathology provoking the blood clotting has been resolved. Chronic, or "long-haul" COVID infections, often demonstrate _**persistent**_ evidence of blood clotting pathology.

In one study, 25% of convalescent COVID patients who were four months past their acute COVID infections demonstrated increased D-dimer levels. Interestingly, these D-dimer elevations were often present when the other common laboratory parameters of abnormal blood clotting had returned to normal.

These other tests included prothrombin time, partial thromboplastin time, fibrinogen level, and platelet count. Inflammation parameters, including C-reactive protein and interleukin-6, typically also had returned to normal (Townsend et al., 2021).

Persistent evidence of blood clotting (increased D-dimer levels) in chronic COVID patients might be a reliable way to determine the persistent presence/production of the COVID spike protein. Another way, discussed below, might be dark field microscopy to look for rouleaux formation of the red blood cells (RBCs).

At the time of the writing of this article, the correlation between an increased D-dimer level and rouleaux formation of the RBCs remains to be determined. Certainly, the presence of both should trigger the greatest of concern for the development of significant chronic COVID and post-COVID vaccination complications.

Is Persistent Spike Protein the Culprit?

Spike proteins are the spear-like appendages attached to and completely surrounding the central core of the COVID virus, giving the virion somewhat of a porcupine-like appearance.

Upon binding to the angiotensin converting enzyme 2 (ACE2) receptors on the cell membranes of the target cells, dissolving enzymes are released that then permit entry of the complete COVID virus into the cytoplasm, where replication of the virus can ensue (Belouzard et al., 2012; Shang et al., 2020).

Concern has been raised regarding the dissemination of the spike protein throughout the body after vaccination.

Rather than staying localized at the injection site in order to provoke the immune response and nothing more, spike protein presence has been detected throughout the body of some vaccinated individuals.

Furthermore, it appears that some of the circulating spike proteins simply bind the ACE2 receptors without entering the cell, inducing an autoimmune response to the entire cell-spike protein entity.

Depending on the cell type that binds the spike protein, any of a number of autoimmune medical conditions can result.

While the underlying pathology remains to be completely defined, one explanation for the problems with thrombotic tendencies and other symptoms seen with chronic COVID and post-vaccination patients relates directly to the persistent presence of the spike protein part of the coronavirus.

Some reports assert that the spike protein can continue to be produced after the initial binding to the ACE2 receptors and entry into some of the cells that it initially targets.

The clinical pictures of chronic COVID and post-vaccine toxicity appear very similar, and both are likely due to this continued presence, and body-wide dissemination, of the spike protein (Mendelson et al., 2020; Aucott and Rebman, 2021; Levy, 2021; Raveendran, 2021).

Although they are found on many different types of cells throughout the body, the ACE2 receptors on the epithelial cells lining the airways are the first targets of the COVID virus upon initial encounter when inhaled (Hoffman et al., 2020).

Furthermore, the concentration of these receptors is especially high on lung alveolar epithelial cells, further causing the lung tissue to be disproportionately targeted by the virus (Alifano et al., 2020).

Unchecked, this avid receptor binding and subsequent viral replication inside the lung cells leads directly to low blood oxygen levels and the adult respiratory distress syndrome [ARDS] (Batah and Fabro, 2021).

Eventually there is a surge of intracellular oxidation known as the cytokine storm, and death from respiratory failure results (Perrotta et al., 2020; Saponaro et al., 2020; Hu et al., 2021).

COVID, Vaccination, and Oxidative Stress

Although some people have prompt and clear-cut negative side effects after COVID vaccination, many appear to do well and feel completely fine after their vaccinations. Is this an assurance that no harm was done, or will be done, by the vaccine in such individuals?

Some striking anecdotal evidence suggests otherwise, while also indicating that there exist good options for optimal protection against side effects in both the short- and long-term.

Under conditions of inflammation and systemically increased oxidative stress, red blood cells (RBCs) can aggregate to varying degrees, sometimes sticking together like stacks of coins with branching of the stacks seen when the stickiness is maximal. This is known as "rouleaux formation" of the RBCs (Samsel and Perelson, 1984).

When this rouleaux formation is pronounced, increased blood viscosity (thickness) is seen, and there is increased resistance to the normal, unimpeded flow of blood, especially in the microcirculation (Sevick and Jain, 1989; Kesmarky et al., 2008; Barshtein et al., 2020; Sloop et al., 2020).

With regard to the smallest capillaries through which the blood must pass, it needs to be noted that individual RBCs literally need to fold slightly to pass from the arterial to the venous side, as the capillary diameter at its narrowest point is actually less than the diameter of a normal RBC, or erythrocyte.

It is clear that any aggregation of the RBCs, as is seen with rouleaux formation, will increase resistance to normal blood flow, and it will be more pronounced as the caliber of the blood vessel decreases.

Not surprisingly, rouleaux formation of the RBCs is also associated with an impaired ability of the blood to optimally transport oxygen, which notably is another feature of COVID spike protein impact (Cicco and Pirrelli, 1999).

Increased RBC aggregation has been observed in a number of different microcirculatory disorders, and it appears to be linked to the pathophysiology in these disorders.

Rouleaux formation is easily visualized directly with dark field microscopy. When available, feedback is immediate, and there is no need to wait for a laboratory to process a test specimen.

It is a reliable indicator of abnormal RBC stickiness and increased blood viscosity, typically elevating the erythrocyte sedimentation test (ESR), an acute phase reactant test that consistently elevates along with C-reactive protein in a setting of generalized increased oxidative stress throughout the body (Lewi and Clarke, 1954; Ramsay and Lerman, 2015).

As such, it can never be dismissed as an incidental and insignificant finding, especially in the setting of a symptom-free individual post-vaccination appearing to be normal and presumably free of body-wide increased inflammation and oxidative stress.

States of advanced degrees of increased systemic oxidative stress, as is often seen in cancer patients, can also display rouleaux formation among circulating neoplastic cells and not just the RBCs (Cho, 2011).

Rouleaux Formation Post-COVID Vaccination

The dark field blood examinations seen below come from a 62-year-old female who had received the COVID vaccination roughly 60 days earlier. The first picture reveals mild rouleaux formation of the blood. After a sequence of six autohemotherapy ozone passes, the second picture shows a completely normal appearance of the RBCs.

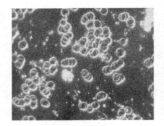 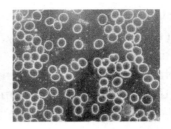

A second patient, a young adult male who received his vaccination 15 days earlier without any side effects noted and feeling completely well at the time, had the dark field examination of his blood performed.

This first examination seen below revealed severe rouleaux formations of the RBCs with extensive branching, appearing to literally involve all of the RBCs visualized in an extensive review of multiple different microscopic fields.

He then received one 400 ml ozonated saline infusion followed by a 15,000 mg infusion of vitamin C. The second picture reveals a complete and immediate resolution of the rouleaux formation seen on the first examination. Furthermore, the normal appearance of the RBCs was still seen 15 days later, giving some reassurance that the therapeutic infusions had some durability, and possibly permanency, in their positive impact.

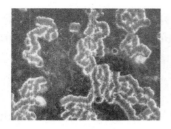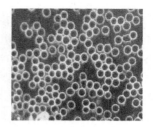

A third adult who received the vaccination 30 days earlier also had severe rouleaux formation on her dark field examination, and this was also completely resolved after the ozonated saline infusion followed by the vitamin C infusion. Of note, similar abnormal dark field microscopy findings were found in other individuals following Pfizer, Moderna, or Johnson & Johnson COVID vaccinations.

Preventing and Treating Chronic COVID and COVID Vaccine Complications

In addition to the mechanisms already discussed by which the spike protein can inflict damage, it appears the spike protein itself is significantly toxic. Such intrinsic toxicity (ability to cause the oxidation of biomolecules) combined with the apparent ability of the spike protein to replicate itself like a complete virus greatly increases the amount of toxic damage that can potentially be inflicted.

A potent toxin is bad enough, but one that can replicate and increase its quantity inside the body after the initial encounter represents a unique challenge among toxins.

And if the mechanism of replication can be sustained indefinitely, the long-term challenge to staying healthy can eventually become insurmountable.

Nevertheless, this toxicity also allows it to be effectively targeted by high enough doses of the ultimate antitoxin, vitamin C, as discussed above. And even the continued production of spike protein can be neutralized by a daily multi-gram dosing of vitamin C, which is an excellent way to support optimal long-term health, anyway.

As was noted in an earlier article (Levy, 2021), there appear to be multiple ways to deal with spike protein effectively.

The approaches to preventing and treating chronic COVID and COVID vaccine complications are similar, except that it would appear that a completely normal D-dimer blood test combined with a completely normal dark field examination of the blood could give the reassurance that the therapeutic goal has been achieved.

Until more data is accumulated on these approaches, it is probably advisable, if possible, to periodically reconfirm the normalcy of both the D-dimer blood test and the dark field blood examination to help assure that no new spike protein synthesis has resumed.

This is particularly important since some patients who are clinically normal and symptom-free following COVID infection have been found to have the COVID virus persist in the fecal matter for an extended period of time (Chen et al., 2020; Patel et al., 2020; Zuo et al., 2020).

Any significant immune challenge or new pathogen exposure facilitating a renewed surge of COVID virus replication could result in a return of COVID symptoms in such persons if the virus cannot be completely eliminated from the body.

Suggested Protocol (to be coordinated with the guidance of your chosen health care provider):

1. For individuals who are post-vaccination or symptomatic with chronic COVID, vitamin C should be optimally dosed, and it should be kept at a high but lesser dose daily indefinitely.

- Ideally, an initial intravenous administration of 25 to 75 grams of vitamin C should be given depending on body size. Although one infusion would likely resolve the symptoms and abnormal blood examination, several more infusions can be given if feasible over the next few days.

- An option that would likely prove to be sufficient and would be much more readily available to larger numbers of patients would be one or more rounds of vitamin C given as a 7.5 gram IV push over roughly 10 minutes, avoiding the need for a complete intravenous infusion setup, a prolonged time in a clinic, and substantially greater expense (Riordan-Clinic-IVC-Push-Protocol, 10.16.14.pdf).

- Additionally, or alternatively if IV is not available, 5 grams of liposome-encapsulated vitamin C (livonlabs.com) can be given daily for at least a week.

- When none of the above three options are readily available, a comparable positive clinical impact will be seen with the proper supplementation of regular forms of oral vitamin C as sodium ascorbate or ascorbic acid. Either of these can be taken daily in three divided doses approaching bowel tolerance after the individual determines their own unique needs (additional information, see Levy, vitamin C Guide in References; Cathcart, 1981).

- An excellent way to support any or all of the above measures for improving vitamin C levels in the body is now available and very beneficial clinically. A supplemental polyphenol that appears to help many to overcome the epigenetic defect preventing the internal synthesis of vitamin C in the liver can be taken once daily. This supplement also appears to provide the individual with the ability to produce and release even greater amounts of vitamin C directly into the blood in the face of infection and other sources of oxidative stress (formula216.com).

2. Hydrogen peroxide (HP) nebulization (Levy, 2021, free eBook) is an antiviral and synergistic partner with vitamin C, and it is especially important in dealing with acute or chronic COVID, or with post-COVID vaccination issues. As noted above, the COVID virus can persist in the stool. In such cases, a chronic pathogen colonization (CPC) of COVID in the throat continually supplying virus that is swallowed into the gut is likely present as well, even when the patient seems to be clinically normal. This will commonly be the case when specific viral eradication measures were not taken during the clinical course of the COVID infection. HP nebulization will clear out this CPC, which will stop the continued seeding of the COVID virus in the gut and stool as well. Different nebulization approaches are discussed in the eBook.

3. When available, ozonated saline and/or ozone autohemotherapy infusions are excellent. Conceivably, this approach alone might suffice to knock out the spike protein presence, but the vitamin C and HP nebulization approaches will also improve and maintain health in general. Ultraviolet blood irradiation and hyperbaric oxygen therapy will likely achieve the same therapeutic effect if available.

4. Ivermectin, hydroxychloroquine, and chloroquine are especially important in preventing new binding of the spike protein to the ACE2 receptors that need to be bound in order for either the spike protein alone or for the entire virus to gain entry into the target cells (Lehrer and Rheinstein, 2020; Wang et al., 2020; Eweas et al., 2021). These agents also appear to have the ability to directly bind up any circulating spike protein before it binds any ACE2 receptors (Fantini et al., 2020; Sehailia and Chemat, 2020; Saha and Raihan, 2021). When the ACE2 receptors are already bound, the COVID virus cannot enter the cell (Pillay, 2020). These three agents also serve as ionophores that promote intracellular accumulation of zinc that is needed to kill/inactivate any intact virus particles that might still be present.

5. Many other positive nutrients, vitamins, and minerals are supportive of defeating the spike protein, but they should not be used to the exclusion of the above, especially the combination of highly-dosed vitamin C and HP nebulization.

Recap

As the pandemic continues, there is an increasing number of chronic COVID patients and post-COVID vaccination patients with a number of different symptoms. Furthermore, there is an increasing number of vaccinated individuals who still end up contracting a COVID infection. This is resulting in a substantial amount of morbidity and mortality around the world.

The presence and persistence of the COVID spike protein, along with the chronic colonization of the COVID virus itself in the aerodigestive tract as well as in the lower gut, appear to be major reasons for illness in this group of patients.

Persistent elevation of D-dimer protein in the blood and the presence of rouleaux formation of the RBCs, especially when advanced in degree, appear to be reliable markers of persistent spike protein-related illness.

The measures noted above, particular the vitamin C and HP nebulization, should result in the disappearance of the D-dimer in the blood while normalizing the appearance of the RBCs examined with dark field microscopy.

Even though new research is taking place daily that may modify therapeutic recommendations, it appears that taking the measures to eliminate D-dimer from the blood and to maintain a consistently normal morphological appearance of the blood is a very practical and efficient way to curtail the ongoing morbidity and mortality secondary to the persistent spike protein presence seen in chronic COVID and in post-COVID vaccination patients.

There are many vaccinated individuals who feel well yet remain cautious about potential future side effects, and who really have no easy access to D-dimer testing or dark field examination of their blood. Such persons can follow a broad-spectrum supplementation regimen featuring vitamin C, magnesium chloride, vitamin D, zinc, and a good multivitamin/multimineral supplement free of iron, copper, and calcium.

Periodic but regular HP nebulization should be included as well. This regimen will offer good spike protein protection while optimizing long-term health. Furthermore, such a long-term supplementation regimen is advisable regardless of how much of the protocol discussed above is followed.

OMNS Contributing Editor Dr. Thomas E. Levy is board certified in internal medicine and cardiology. He is also an attorney, admitted to the bar in Colorado and in the District of Columbia.

The views presented in this article are the author's and not necessarily those of all members of the Orthomolecular Medicine News Service Editorial Review Board.)

This article was provided by the Orthomolecular Medicine News Service. For a free subscription go to orthomolecular.org/subscribe and to view the OMNS archives visit orthomolecular.org/resources

1

Alifano M, Alifano P, Forgez P, Iannelli A (2020) Renin-angiotensin system at the heart of the COVID-19 pandemic. Biochemie 174:30-33. PMID: 32305506

2

Aucott J, Rebman A (2021) Long-haul COVID: heed the lessons from other infection-triggered illnesses. Lancet 397:967-968. PMID: 33684352

3

Barshtein G, Waynblum D, Yedgar S (2020) Kinetics of linear rouleaux formation studied by visual monitoring of red cell dynamic organization. Biophysical Journal 78:2470-2474. PMID: 10777743

4

Batah S, Fabro A (2021) Pulmonary pathology of ARDS in COVID-19: a pathological review for clinicians. Respiratory Medicine 176:106239. PMID: 33246294

5

Belouzard S, Millet J, Licitra B, Whittaker G (2012) Mechanisms of coronavirus cell entry mediated by the viral spike protein. Viruses 4:1011-1033. PMID: 22816037

6

Biswas S, Thakur V, Kaur P et al. (2021) Blood clots in COVID-19 patients: simplifying the curious mystery. Medical Hypotheses 146:110371. PMID: 33223324

7

Carli G, Nichele I, Ruggeri M, Barra S, Tosetto A (2021) Deep vein thrombosis (DVT) occurring shortly after the second dose of mRNA SARS-CoV-2 vaccine. Internal and Emergency Medicine 16:803-804. PMID: 336876791

8

Cathcart R (1981) Vitamin C, titrating to bowel tolerance, anascorbemia, and acute induced scurvy. Medical Hypotheses 7:1359-1376. PMID: 7321921

9

Chen Y, Chen L, Deng Q et al. (2020) The presence of SARS-CoV-2 RNA I the feces of COVID-19 patients. Journal of Medical Virology 92:833-840. PMID: 32243607

10

Cho S (2011) Plasma cell leukemia with rouleaux formation involving neoplastic cells and RBC. The Korean Journal of Hematology 46:152. PMID: 22065968

11

Cicci G, Pirrelli A (1999) Red blood cell (RBC) deformability, RBC aggregability and tissue oxygenation in hypertension. Clinical Hemorheology and Microcirculation 21:169-177. PMID: 10711739

12

Eweas A, Alhossary A, Abdel-Moneim A (2021) Molecular docking reveals ivermectin and remdesivir as potential repurposed drugs against SARS-CoV-2. Frontiers in Microbiology 11:592908. PMID: 33746908

13

Fantini J, Di Scala C, Chahinian H, Yahi N (2020) Structural and molecular modelling studies reveal a new mechanism of action of chloroquine and hydroxychloroquine against SARS-CoV-2 infection. International Journal of Antimicrobial Agents 55:105960. PMID: 32251731

14

Favaloro E (2021) Laboratory testing for suspected COVID-19 vaccine-induced (immune) thrombotic thrombocytopenia. International Journal of Laboratory Hematology 43:559-570. PMID: 34138513

15

Hoffman M, Kleine-Weber H, Schroeder S et al. (2020) SARS-CoV-2 entry depends on ACE 2 and TMPRSS2 and is blocked by a clinically proven protease inhibitor. Cell 181:271-280. PMID: 32142651

16

Hu B, Huang S, Yin L (2021) The cytokine storm and COVID-19. Journal of Medical Virology 93:250-256. PMID: 32592501

17

Iba T, Levy J, Levi M et al. (2020) Coagulopathy of coronavirus disease 2019. Critical Care Medicine 48:1358-1364. PMID: 32467443

18

Iba T, Levy J, Warkentin T (2021) Recognizing vaccine-induced immune thrombotic thrombocytopenia. Critical Care Medicine [Online ahead of print]. PMID: 34259661

19

Kesmarky G, Kenyeres P, Rabai M, Toth K (2008) Plasma viscosity: a forgotten variable. Clinical Hemorheology and Microcirculation 39:243-246. PMID: 18503132

20

Lehrer S, Rheinstein P (2020) Ivermectin docks to the SARS-CoV-2 spike receptor-binding domain attached to ACE 2. In Vivo 34:3023-3026. PMID: 32871846

21

Levy T Guide-to-Optimal-Admin-of-IVC-10-18-2021.pdf

22

Levy T (2002) Curing the Incurable. Vitamin C, Infectious Diseases, and Toxins Henderson, NV: MedFox Publishing

23

Levy T (2019) Magnesium, Reversing Disease Chapter 12, Henderson, NV: MedFox Publishing

24

Levy T (2021) Resolving "Long-Haul COVID" and vaccine toxicity: neutralizing the spike protein.
Orthomolecular Medicine News Service June 21, 2021.
orthomolecular.org/resources/omns

25
Levy T (2021) Rapid Virus Recovery: No need to live in fear! Henderson, NV: MedFox Publishing. Free eBook download (English or Spanish) available at rvr.medfoxpub.com

26
Lewi S, Clarke K (1954) Rouleaux formation intensity and E.S.R. British Medical Journal 2:336-338. PMID: 13182211

27
Lundstrom K, Barh D, Uhal B et al. (2021) COVID-19 vaccines and thrombosis-roadblock or dead-end street? Biomolecules 11:1020. PMID: 34356644

28
Mendelson M, Nel J, Blumberg L et al. (2020) Long-COVID: an evolving problem with an extensive impact. South African Medical Journal 111:10-12. PMID: 33403997

29
Naymagon L, Zubizarreta N, Feld J et al. (2020) Admission D-dimer levels, D-dimer trends, and outcomes in COVID-19. Thrombosis Research 196:99-105. PMID: 32853982

30
Paliogiannis P, Mangoni A, Dettori P et al. (2020) D-dimer concentrations and COVID-19 severity: a systematic review and meta-analysis. Frontiers in Public Health 8:432. PMID: 32903841

31

Patel K, Patel P, Vunnam R et al. (2020) Gastrointestinal, hepatobiliary, and pancreatic manifestations of COVID-19. Journal of Clinical Virology 128:104386. PMID: 32388469

32

Perricone C, Ceccarelli F, Nesher G et al. (2014) Immune thrombocytopenic purpura (ITP) associated with vaccinations: a review of reported cases. Immunologic Research 60:226-235. PMID: 25427992

33

Perrotta F, Matera M, Cazzola M, Bianco A (2020) Severe respiratory SARS-CoV2 infection: does ACE2 receptor matter? Respiratory Medicine 168:105996. PMID: 32364961

34

Perry R, Tamborska A, Singh B et al. (2021) Cerebral venous thrombosis after vaccination against COVID-19 in the UK: a multicentre cohort study. Lancet Aug 6. Online ahead of print. PMID: 34370972

35

Pillay T (2020) Gene of the month: the 2019-nCoV/SARS-CoV-2 novel coronavirus spike protein. Journal of Clinical Pathology 73:366-369. PMID: 32376714

36
Ramsay E, Lerman M (2015) How to use the erythrocyte sedimentation rate in paediatrics. Archives of Disease in Childhood. Education and Practice Edition 100:30-36. PMID: 25205237

37
Raveendran A (2021) Long COVID-19: Challenges in the diagnosis and proposed diagnostic criteria. Diabetes & Metabolic Syndrome: Clinical Research & Reviews 15:145-146. PMID: 33341598

38
Rostami M, Mansouritorghabeh H (2020) D-dimer level in COVID-19 infection: a systematic review. Expert Review of Hematology 13:1265-1275. PMID: 32997543

39
Saha J, Raihan M (2021) The binding mechanism of ivermectin and levosalbutamol with spike protein of SARS-CoV-2. Structural Chemistry Apr 12. Online ahead of print. PMID: 33867777

40
Samsel R, Perelson A (1984) Kinetics of rouleau formation. II. Reversible reactions. Biophysical Journal 45:805-824. PMID: 6426540

41

Saponaro F, Rutigliano G, Sestito S et al. (2020) ACE 2 in the era of SARS-CoV-2: controversies and novel perspectives. Frontiers in Molecular Biosciences 7:588618. PMID: 33195436

42

Scully M, Singh D, Lown R et al. (2021) Pathologic antibodies to platelet factor 4 after ChAdOx1 nCoV-19 vaccination. The New England Journal of Medicine 384:2202-2211. PMID: 33861525

43

Sehailia M, Chemat S (2021) Antimalarial-agent artemisinin and derivatives portray more potent binding of Lys353 and Lys31-binding hotspots of SARS-CoV-2 spike protein than hydroxychloroquine: potential repurposing of artenimol for COVID-19. Journal of Biomolecular Structure & Dynamics 39:6184-6194. PMID: 32696720

44

Sevick E, Jain R (1989) Viscous resistance to blood flow in solid tumors: effect of hemocrit on intratumor blood viscosity. Cancer Research 49:3513-3519. PMID: 2731173

45

Shang J, Wan Y, Luo C et al. (2020) Cell entry mechanisms of SARS-CoV-2. Proceedings of the National Academy of Sciences of the United States of America 117:11727-11734. PMID: 32376634

46

Sloop G, De Mast Q, Pop G et al. (2020) The role of blood viscosity in infectious diseases. Cureus 12:e7090. PMID: 32226691

47

Subramaniam S, Scharrer I (2018) Procoagulant activity during viral infections. Frontiers in Bioscience 23:1060-1081. PMID: 28930589

48

Thaler J, Ay C, Gleixner K et al. (2021) Successful treatment of vaccine-induced prothrombotic immune thrombocytopenia (VIPIT). Journal of Thrombosis and Haemostasis 19:1819-1822. PMID: 33877735

49

Townsend L, Fogarty H, Dyer A et al. (2021) Prolonged elevation of D-dimer levels in convalescent COVID-19 patients is independent of the acute phase response. Journal of Thrombosis and Haemostasis 19:1064-1070. PMID: 33587810

50

Wang N, Han S, Liu R et al. (2020) Chloroquine and hydroxychloroquine as ACE2 blockers to inhibit viropexis of 2019-nCoV spike pseudotyped virus. Phytomedicine: International Journal of Phytotherapy and Phytopharmacology 79:153333. PMID: 32920291

51

Zhang S, Liu Y, Want X et al. (2021) SARS-Cov-2 binds platelet ACE2 to enhance thrombosis in COVID-19. Journal of Hematology & Oncology 13:120. PMID: 32887634

53

Zuo T, Zhang F, Lui G et al. (2020) Alterations in gut microbiota of patients with COVID-19 during time of hospitalization. Gastroenterology 159:944-955. PMID: 32442562

04

Online Resources

Chapter Eighteen
Patient Advocacy Groups

Unique to this pandemic is the creation and role of patient advocacy groups in identifying persistent symptoms and influencing research and clinical attention.

Surveys conducted by these groups have helped identify persistent symptoms such as brain fog, fatigue, and body aches as essential components of long haul Covid.

NBC News reports that Survivor Corps is one of the most popular among Facebook groups, but more than 4.5 million people have joined around 4,000 Covid-19 supports groups in the U.S. Medical authorities warn against taking advice found in such groups, but some doctors find they can be helpful for some patients and even for doctors seeking to conduct surveys and gather information.[104]

Additionally, they have been instrumental in highlighting the persistence of symptoms in patients with mild-to-moderate disease who did not require hospitalization.

Active engagement with these patient advocacy groups, many of whom identify as long haulers, is crucial.

ONLINE SUPPORT RESOURCES

U.S/CANADA COVID WEBSITES

Covid Long Haulers Treatment Program *(Incell DX)*

C19 Recovery Awareness *(United States)*

Covid Long-Haul Canada *(Canada)*

Canadian Covid Care Alliance

Long Covid Canada

Covid Care Group

Survivor Corps

Long-Covid Alliance

Patient Advocate Foundation

The Advocacy Exchange

DISABILITY LEGAL RESOURCES

Kantor & Kantor Law Firm *(United States)*

U.K.& E.U.COVID WEBSITES

Covid-19 Collective Recovery *(Asthma UK & British Lung Foundation (English)*

The Royal Society of Medicine Covid-19 Learning Hub

Long Covid Kids

Covid-19 Persistente *(Spanish)*

Apuakoronaan.fi *(Finnish)*

Long Covid Scotland *(Scotland)*

Soutien/Revue de Presse Covid-19 *(French)*

Corona Longplein *(Dutch)*

Ook Dit Is Covid *(Dutch)*

Post-Covid Gemeenschap*(Dutch)*

Long Covid Deutschland **(German***)*

FACEBOOK

Long Haul Covid Fighters (Onset Before April 1st, 2020)
Long Haul Covid Fighters (Onset Before April 1st, 2020 Round 2
Long Covid Support Group
Long Haul Covid Fighters Medical & Scientific Collaboration
Covid Long Haulers Support Group Canada
Long Covid Scotland Action Group
Corona ervaringen en langdurige klachten! (*Dutch*)
Malades et Gueris du Coronavirus (*French*)
COVID-19 Langzeitbeschwerden (*German*)
Corona patiënten met langdurige klachten (Vlaanderen) (*Dutch*)
Koronaviruksen saaneet ja oireilevat keskusteluryhmä (*Finnish*)
Covid-19 témoignages : maladie, guérison, astuces et soutien (*French*)
Long Covid ACTS (**Spanish**)

TWITTER

Worldwide #LongCovid
Brasil Long Covid BR
Finland #Koronaoire
France Long Covid France #apresj20
Germany #MitCoronaLeben #Langzeit
Italy #Covidpersistenteitalia
Japan #長期微熱組
Netherlands Long COVID Netherlands
New Zealand LongCovidNZ #LongCovidNZ
Scotland Long Covid Scotland

REDDIT

Covid-19 Positive Support

SLACK

Body Politic Covid-19 Support Group

CONCLUSION

Roadmap to Recovery describes the developments that took place leading up to long haul Covid. It describes how Covid-19 became a global pandemic and in addition to infecting millions of people around the globe, resulting in the death of many, it has also left many survivors with long haul Covid.

It did not seem to matter whether you had a serious case of Covid-19 or a mild one, whether you were hospitalized or not, whether you had comorbidities or not, whether you were young and healthy, long haul Covid could affect anyone.

The Roadmap goes on to report that long haul Covid represents a serious challenge to the existing healthcare system. The existing system with its organ focused approach is ill-suited to deal with a chronic disease like long haul.

It points out that more attention should be focused on the nutritional health of the population, bolstering the body's natural immune system and starting early treatment rather than waiting for individuals to get sick enough to be admitted to the hospital.

The Roadmap identifies some of the innovative and complementary treatments that are being used to alleviate the symptoms that afflict long haul sufferers. The Roadmap points out that the ball is now in the long haulers' court.

The chapter "Choosing Your Own Path" details the choices a long hauler has to make in determining their own path to recovery. You now have the Roadmap It is up to you to take action, either with your current healthcare provider, or if necessary, to find a new one.

Included is a listing of patient advocacy groups from around the world. These groups can offer support and allow for the sharing of information. They can be an invaluable resource for anyone with long haul Covid or for someone who wants to help someone with long haul Covid.

My hope is that you will have found this book informative and are able to take some action to alleviate your symptoms. If so, then my purpose in writing this book will have been fulfilled.

If you found the information helpful, please leave a review on Amazon. Letting others know you found this information important will increase the visibility of the book. It will help those suffering from long haul Covid find this book. I look forward to reading your review.

GHR

VOL. 01/2021   PUBLISIHING NEWS

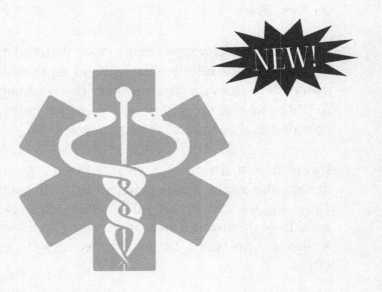

NEW!

THIRTEEN DIFFERENT
MODALITIES
INCLUDING LINKS
TO THEIR
PRACTITIONERS.

A Comprehensive Guide
to Non-Conventional
Treatments for Chronic
Diseases

JDGOODMAN.CA/ROADMAP-TO-RECOVERY

ACKNOWLEGMENTS

This book, like many other publications, is the result of the efforts of many people.

First, and foremost, are the doctors, researchers, and scientists who, when faced with the Covid-19 pandemic and its after-effect, long haul Covid, rose to the occasion and developed treatments and protocols that benefited their patients and all of humanity.

This book contains a brief summary of their published research and clinical practice.

The sufferers of long haul Covid have been a major catalyst for my publishing this book. I gratefully acknowledge the contribution made by the long haulers' stories in this book – Morgan Stephens, Heather-Elizabeth Brown and Amanda Thebe.

Their stories bring to life what all the facts and figures cannot describe – the debilitating, terrorizing effects of long haul Covid. I am also grateful to their publishers, CNN and Remedy Health Media , for permission to reprint their stories.

My research showed there are ways to treat this illness and they are not easily found.

This book aims to make it easier to discover the various treatments that are being utilized to combat long haul Covid.

Thanks to my wife, Laurie De Camillis, who joined with me to begin our publishing business, encouraged me to write a book to share the information that I had collected over many months and who, while writing her own book, made the time to help me, every step of the way.

My Historian, Dustin Galer, Ph.D. who took my pages and pages of research and turned them into a readable narrative without compromising the integrity of the material.

Jacqueline Carlisle who formatted our thousands of words into a beautiful book and enclosed it with a stunning cover.

Dustin Galer, Ph.D..

Book design by Jacqueline Carlisle

ABOUT THE AUTHOR

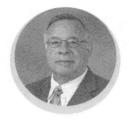

Jeffrey D Goodman has a Doctorate in Education from the University of Massachusetts.

He has been a university professor and has served as the Director of Professional Development for The Ontario Dental Association.

He also suffers from chronic kidney disease. He spent years journeying through the traditional healthcare system and networks of alternative medicine providers as he learned more about how to live with his condition.

His personal experiences taught him about the many challenges facing other chronic disease sufferers, which developed into a passion for educating and empowering others like him.

This is his first book in an anticipated series dedicated to educating the public about chronic disease.

REFERENCES

[1]
*COVID 'Long Haulers': Long-Term Effects of COVID-19. 2021
Retrieved 8 September 2021, from*

hopkinsmedicine.org/health/conditions-and-
diseases/coronavirus/covid-long-haulers-long-term-
effects-of-covid19

[2]
*The Long Haul: Forging a Path through the Lingering Effects
of COVID-19 | 2021 Congressional Testimony from
CDC. (2021). Retrieved 8 September 2021, from
https://www.cdc.gov/washington/testimony/2021/t2021042
8.htm*

[3]
*COVID-19 and Your Health. (2020).
Retrieved 9 September 2021, from*
cdc.gov/coronavirus/2019-ncov/long-term-effects.html

[4]
*COVID-19 and Your Health. (2020).
Retrieved 8 September 2021, from*
cdc.gov/coronavirus/2019-ncov/long-term-effects.html

[5]
*Long COVID FAQs — Survivor Corps. (2021).
Retrieved 9 September 2021, from*
survivorcorps.com/long-covid-faqs

[6] Aucott, J., & Rebman, A. (2021). Long-haul COVID: heed the lessons from other infection-triggered illnesses. *The Lancet, 397*(10278), 967-968. DOI: 10.1016/s0140-6736(21)00446-3.

[7] *Healthcare Workers*. (2020).
Retrieved 20 September 2021, from
cdc.gov/coronavirus/2019-ncov/hcp/clinical-care/post-covid-conditions.html

[8] Davis, H., Assaf, G., McCorkell, L., Wei, H., Low, R., & Re'em, Y. et al. (2021). *Characterizing long COVID in an international cohort: 7 months of symptoms and their impact. Eclinicalmedicine, 38*, 101019.
DOI: 10.1016/j.eclinm.2021.101019

[9] *Newsroom | FAIR Health*. (2021). Retrieved
9 September 2021, from
fairhealth.org/press-release/nineteen-percent-of-asymptomatic-covid-19-patients-develop-long-haul-covid

[10] Al-Aly, Z., Xie, Y., & Bowe, B. (2021). *High-dimensional characterization of post-acute sequelae of COVID-19. Nature, 594*(7862), 259-264. DOI: 10.1038/s41586-021-03553-9.

[11] *The Long Haul: Forging a Path through the Lingering Effects of COVID-19 | 2021 Congressional Testimony from CDC*. (2021). Retrieved 9 September 2021, from
https://www.cdc.gov/washington/testimony/2021/t20210428.htm

[12] *Ibid; COVID-19 and Your Health. (2020). Retrieved 9 September 2021, from* https://www.cdc.gov/coronavirus/2019-ncov/long-term-effects.html *; Mokhtari, T., Hassani, F., Ghaffari, N., Ebrahimi, B., Yarahmadi, A., & Hassanzadeh, G. (2020). COVID-19 and multiorgan failure: A narrative review on potential mechanisms. Journal Of Molecular Histology, 51(6), 613–628. doi: 10.1007/s10735-020-09915-3.*

[13] Ibid;

[14] *COVID 'Long Haulers': Long-Term Effects of COVID-19. (2021). Retrieved 9 September 2021, from* https://www.hopkinsmedicine.org/health/conditions-and-diseases/coronavirus/covid-long-haulers-long-term-effects-of-covid19.

[15] *COVID-19 (coronavirus): Long-term effects. (2021). Retrieved 10 September 2021, from* https://www.mayoclinic.org/diseases-conditions/coronavirus/in-depth/coronavirus-long-term-effects/art-20490351.

[16] *COVID 'Long Haulers': Long-Term Effects of COVID-19. (2021). Retrieved 10 September 2021, from* https://www.hopkinsmedicine.org/health/conditions-and-diseases/coronavirus/covid-long-haulers-long-term-effects-of-covid19

[17] *COVID-19 study: Prevalence of unusual symptoms in older adults | Northwell Health. (2021). Retrieved 10 September 2021, from https://feinstein.northwell.edu/news/the-latest/covid-19-study-prevalence-of-unusual-symptoms-in-older-adults*

[18] *UC Davis Health, P. (2021). Studies show long-haul COVID-19 afflicts 1 in 4 COVID-19 patients, regardless of severity. Retrieved 8 September 2021, from https://health.ucdavis.edu/health-news/newsroom/studies-show-long-haul-covid-19-afflicts-1-in-4-covid-19-patients-regardless-of-severity/2021/03*

[19] *Inside 'post-Covid' clinics: How specialized centers are trying to treat long-haulers. (2021). Retrieved 9 September 2021, from https://www.nbcnews.com/health/health-news/inside-post-covid-clinics-how-specialized-centers-are-trying-treat-n1258879*

[20] *Greenhalgh, T., Knight, M., A'Court, C., Buxton, M., & Husain, L. (2020). Management of post-acute covid-19 in primary care. BMJ, m3026. DOI: 10.1136/BMJ.m3026*

[21] *COVID 'Long Haulers': Long-Term Effects of COVID-19. (2021). Retrieved 8 September 2021, from https://www.hopkinsmedicine.org/health/conditions-and-diseases/coronavirus/covid-long-haulers-long-term-effects-of-covid19*

[22] *COVID-19 (coronavirus): Long-term effects. (2021). Retrieved 8 September 2021, from* https://www.mayoclinic.org/diseases-conditions/coronavirus/in-depth/coronavirus-long-term-effects/art-20490351

[23] *COVID 'Long Haulers': Long-Term Effects of COVID-19. (2021). Retrieved 9 September 2021, from* https://www.hopkinsmedicine.org/health/conditions-and-diseases/coronavirus/covid-long-haulers-long-term-effects-of-covid19.

[24] *Half of COVID-19 patients report symptoms after 12 weeks, says new PHAC review. Retrieved 9 September 2021, from* https://ca.news.yahoo.com/half-covid-19-patients-report-172305174.html

[25] *Newsroom | FAIR Health. (2021). Retrieved 9 September 2021, from* https://www.fairhealth.org/press-release/nineteen-percent-of-asymptomatic-covid-19-patients-develop-long-haul-covid

[26] *COVID-19 and Your Health. (2020). Retrieved 9 September 2021, from* https://www.cdc.gov/coronavirus/2019-ncov/long-term-effects.html

[27] *COVID-19 and Your Health. (2020). Retrieved 9 September 2021, from https://www.cdc.gov/coronavirus/2019-ncov/long-term-effects.html*

[28] *COVID 'Long Haulers': Long-Term Effects of COVID-19. (2021). Retrieved 9 September 2021, from https://www.hopkinsmedicine.org/health/conditions-and-diseases/coronavirus/covid-long-haulers-long-term-effects-of-covid19*

[29] *Rourke, M. (2021). Unlocking the Mysteries of Long COVID. Retrieved 8 September 2021, from https://www.theatlantic.com/magazine/archive/2021/04/unlocking-the-mysteries-of-long-covid/618076/*

[30] *The Long Haul: Forging a Path through the Lingering Effects of COVID-19 | 2021 Congressional Testimony from CDC. (2021). Retrieved 9 September 2021, from https://www.cdc.gov/washington/testimony/2021/t20210428.htm*

[31] *COVID-19 and Your Health. (2020). Retrieved 9 September 2021, from https://www.cdc.gov/coronavirus/2019-ncov/long-term-effects.html*

[32] *Confronting Our Next National Health Disaster — Long-Haul Covid | NEJM. (2021). New England Journal Of Medicine. Retrieved from* https://www.nejm.org/doi/full/10.1056/NEJMp2109285

[33] *Ibid;*

[34] *Ibid;*

[35] *Yong, E. (2020). Long-Haulers Are Redefining COVID-19. Retrieved 9 September 2021, from* https://www.theatlantic.com/health/archive/2020/08/long-haulers-covid-19-recognition-support-groups-symptoms/615382/

[36] *Dysautonomia: Symptoms, Causes, Types, & How to Live With. (2021). Retrieved 9 September 2021, from* https://my.clevelandclinic.org/health/diseases/6004-dysautonomia

[37] *Rourke, M. (2021). Unlocking the Mysteries of Long COVID. Retrieved 9 September 2021, from* https://www.theatlantic.com/magazine/archive/2021/04/unlocking-the-mysteries-of-long-covid/618076/

[38] *Pomeroy, C. (2021). A Tsunami of Disability Is Coming as a Result of ‘ Long COVID’ Retrieved 9 September 2021, from* https://www.scientificamerican.com/article/a-tsunami-of-disability-is-coming-as-a-result-of-lsquo-long-covid-rsquo

[39] *CDC Has Not Tracked the Comorbidities of the 361 ChilDr.en 17 and Under Who Died of COVID. (2021). Retrieved 13 September 2021, from* https://www.cnsnews.com/article/national/susan-jones/cdc-has-not-tracked-comorbidities-361-children-17-and-under-who-died

[40] *Tsankov, B., Allaire, J., Irvine, M., Lopez, A., Sauvé, L., Vallance, B., & Jacobson, K. (2021). Severe COVID-19 Infection and Pediatric Comorbidities: A Systematic Review and Meta-Analysis. International Journal Of Infectious Diseases, 103, 246-256. DOI: 10.1016/j.ijid.2020.11.163*

[41] *Coronavirus Disease 2019 (COVID-19). (2020). Retrieved 13 September 2021, from* https://www.cdc.gov/coronavirus/2019-ncov/science/science-briefs/sars-cov-2-transmission.html#:~:text=Exposure%20occurs%20in%20three%20principal,hands%20that%20have%20been%20soiled

[42] *Coronavirus Disease 2019 (COVID-19). (2020). Retrieved 13 September 2021, from* https://www.cdc.gov/coronavirus/2019-ncov/science/science-briefs/sars-cov-2-transmission.html?CDC_AA_refVal=https%3A%2F%2Fwww.cdc.gov%2Fcoronavirus%2F2019-ncov%2Fscience%2Fscience-briefs%2Fscientific-brief-sars-cov-2.html

[43] *Ibid;*

[44] *Ibid;*

[45] *COVID-19 and Your Health. (2021). Retrieved 13 September 2021, from https://www.cdc.gov/coronavirus/2019-ncov/prevent-getting-sick/how-covid-spreads.html*

[46] *COVID-19 Vaccination. (2020). Retrieved 13 September 2021, from https://www.cdc.gov/coronavirus/2019-ncov/vaccines/keythingstoknow.html*

[47] *Coronavirus: DOD Response. (2021). Retrieved 13 September 2021, from https://www.defense.gov/Explore/Spotlight/Coronavirus-DOD-Response*

[48] *Emergency Use Authorization for Vaccines Explained. (2020). Retrieved 13 September 2021, from https://www.fda.gov/vaccines-blood-biologics/vaccines/emergency-use-authorization-vaccines-explained*

[49] *FDA Approves First COVID-19 Vaccine. (2021). Retrieved 20 September 2021, from https://www.fda.gov/news-events/press-announcements/fda-approves-first-covid-19-vaccine*

[50] *Coronavirus Disease 2019 (COVID-19). (2020). Retrieved 13 September 2021, from https://www.cdc.gov/coronavirus/2019-ncov/science/science-briefs/sars-cov-2-transmission.html? CDC_AA_refVal=https%3A%2F%2Fwww.cdc.gov%2Fcoronavirus%2F2019-ncov%2Fscience%2Fscience-briefs%2Fscientific-brief-sars-cov-2.html*

[51] *Coronavirus disease 2019 (COVID-19) - Symptoms and causes. (2021). Retrieved 13 September 2021, from https://www.mayoclinic.org/diseases-conditions/coronavirus/symptoms-causes/syc-20479963*

[52] *Prevention and Prophylaxis of SARS-CoV-2 Infection (2021). Retrieved 13 September 2021, from https://www.covid19treatmentguidelines.nih.gov/overview/prevention-of-sars-cov-2/*

[53] *COVID-19 Mythbusters – World Health Organization. (2021). Retrieved 13 September 2021, from https://www.who.int/emergencies/diseases/novel-coronavirus-2019/advice-for-public/myth-busters#supplements*

[54] *Coronavirus Disease 2019 (COVID-19) Treatment Guidelines (2021). Retrieved 13 September 2021, from* https://files.covid19treatmentguidelines.nih.gov/guidelines/covid19treatmentguidelines.pdf

[55] *Lim, Z., Subramaniam, A., Ponnapa Reddy, M., Blecher, G., Kadam, U., & Afroz, A. et al. (2021). Case Fatality Rates for Patients with COVID-19 Requiring Invasive Mechanical Ventilation. A Meta-analysis. American Journal Of Respiratory And Critical Care Medicine, 203(1), 54-66. DOI: 10.1164/rccm.202006-2405oc*

[56] *CDC Studies Show Vaccine Protection Wanes Over Time, Less Effective Against Delta Variant. (2021). Retrieved 13 September 2021, from* https://childrenshealthdefense.org/defender/cdc-vaccine-protection-less-effective-against-delta-variant/

[57] *Having SARS-CoV-2 once confers much greater immunity than a vaccine—but vaccination remains vital. (2021). Retrieved 13 September 2021, from* https://www.science.org/content/article/having-sars-cov-2-once-confers-much-greater-immunity-vaccine-vaccination-remains-vital

[58] *Good news: Mild COVID-19 induces lasting antibody protection | Washington University School of Medicine in St. Louis. (2021). Retrieved 13 September 2021, from* https://medicine.wustl.edu/news/good-news-mild-covid-19-induces-lasting-antibody-protection/

[59] *What is Terrain Theory and Germ Theory?. (2021). Retrieved 13 September 2021, from* https://thefullest.com/2021/03/25/what-is-terrain-theory-and-germ-theory/; *Rethinking our Health Model – Germ Vs Terrain Theory. (2021). Retrieved 13 September 2021, from* https://www.curamedicine.com.au/blog/rethinking-our-health-model-germ-vs-terrain-theory/

[60] *Rethinking our Health Model – Germ Vs Terrain Theory. (2021). Retrieved 13 September 2021, from* https://www.curamedicine.com.au/blog/rethinking-our-health-model-germ-vs-terrain-theory/

[61] *Kostoff RN, Briggs MB, Porter AL, et al. The under-reported role of toxic substance exposures in the COVID-19 pandemic. Food and Chemical Toxicology: An International Journal Published for the British Industrial Biological Research Association. 2020 Nov;145:111687. PMC, E. (2021). Europe PMC. Retrieved 13 September 2021, from* https://europepmc.org/article/MED/32805343

[62] Ibid;

[63] *Lasting immunity found after recovery from COVID-19. (2021). Retrieved 13 September 2021, from* https://www.nih.gov/news-events/nih-research-matters/lasting-immunity-found-after-recovery-covid-19

[64] *A New Roadmap for Treating Disease | Dr. Mark Hyman. (2018). Retrieved 13 September 2021, from* https://Dr.hyman.com/blog/2018/05/16/a-new-roadmap-for-treating-disease/

[65] *The Body Can Heal Itself - Dr William Li. (2019). Retrieved 13 September 2021, from* https://drwilliamli.com/the-body-can-heal-itself/; *An Overview of Immunity (And How to Boost It) - Dr William Li. (2020). Retrieved 13 September 2021, from* https://drwilliamli.com/an-overview-of-immunity-and-how-to-boost-it

[66] *Alan Goldhamer, D. (2010). How Your Body Heals Itself - Center for Nutrition Studies. Retrieved 13 September 2021, from* https://nutritionstudies.org/body-heals/

[67] *Hewison, M. (2011). Vitamin D and immune function: an overview. Proceedings Of The Nutrition Society, 71(1), 50-61. DOI: 10.1017/s0029665111001650*

[68] *Martens, P., Gysemans, C., Verstuyf, A., & Mathieu, C. (2020). Vitamin D's Effect on Immune Function. Nutrients, 12(5), 1248. DOI: 10.3390/nu12051248*

[69] Aranow, C. (2011). Vitamin D and the Immune System. Journal Of Investigative Medicine, 59(6), 881–886. DOI: 10.2310/jim.0b013e31821b8755

[70] J, K., & M, I. (2015). [Current Topics on Vitamin D. The effects of vitamin D on the immune system]. Clinical Calcium, 25(3). Retrieved from https://pubmed.ncbi.nlm.nih.gov/25716808/

[71] Shakoor, H., Feehan, J., Al Dhaheri, A., Ali, H., Platat, C., & Ismail, L. et al. (2021). Immune-boosting role of vitamins D, C, E, zinc, selenium and omega-3 fatty acids: Could they help against COVID-19?. Maturitas, 143, 1–9. DOI: 10.1016/j.maturitas.2020.08.003

[72] Healthcare Workers. (2020). Retrieved 16 September 2021, from https://www.cdc.gov/coronavirus/2019-ncov/hcp/clinical-care/post-covid-management.html

[73] Healthcare Workers. (2020). Retrieved 16 September 2021, from https://www.cdc.gov/coronavirus/2019-ncov/hcp/clinical-care/post-covid-index.html

[74] The study underscores the need for multidisciplinary care for COVID-19 long-haulers Retrieved 17 September 2021, from https://www.dana-farber.org/newsroom/news-releases/2021/study-underscores-need-for-multidisciplinary-care-for-covid-19-long-haulers/

[75] *Inside 'post-Covid' clinics: How specialized centers are trying to treat long-haulers. (2021). Retrieved 17 September 2021, from https://www.nbcnews.com/health/health-news/inside-post-covid-clinics-how-specialized-centers-are-trying-treat-n1258879*

[76] *Programs Help COVID Long Haulers Recover. (2021). Retrieved 17 September 2021, from https://www.webmd.com/lung/news/20210216/programs-help-covid-long-haulers-recover*

[77] *Rourke, M. (2021). Unlocking the Mysteries of Long COVID. Retrieved 17 September 2021, from https://www.theatlantic.com/magazine/archive/2021/04/unlocking-the-mysteries-of-long-covid/618076/*

[78] *EXPOSED, H. (2021). Spike Protein Biomarkers for Adverse Risk - Part 3. Retrieved 17 September 2021, from https://rumble.com/vles5d-spike-protein-biomarkers-for-adverse-risk-part-3.html*

[79] *How to Use Blood Testing to Increase Your Resilience to COVID (2021). Retrieved 17 September 2021, from https://a9134cad-f409-4ff0-9add-f8cc45699c23.filesusr.com/ugd/5e2a5e_47a472382ea74764a6800d51cf899479.pdf*

[80] *Functional Medicine | IFM. (2021). Retrieved 18 September 2021, from https://www.ifm.org/functional-medicine/*

[81] *What is Functional Medicine? (2021).*
Retrieved 18 September 2021, from
https://my.clevelandclinic.org/departments/functional-
medicine/about

[82] *The Functional Medicine Approach to COVID-19: Virus-*
Specific Nutraceutical and Botanical Agents | The Institute for
Functional Medicine. (2021). Retrieved 18 September 2021,
from https://www.ifm.org/news-insights/the-functional-
medicine-approach-to-covid-19-virus-specific-
nutraceutical-and-botanical-agents/

[83] *How to Treat Long-Haul COVID. (2021). Retrieved 18*
September 2021, from
https://experiencelife.lifetime.life/article/how-to-treat-long-
haul-covid/;

[84] *Venkatesan, P. (2021). NICE guideline on long COVID. The*
Lancet Respiratory Medicine, 9(2), 129. doi:
10.1016/s2213-2600(21)00031-x

[85] *About us – FLCCC | Front Line COVID-19 Critical Care Alliance.*
Retrieved 24 September 2021, from
https://covid19criticalcare.com/about/

[86] *The FLCCC Physicians – FLCCC | Front Line COVID-19 Critical*
Care Alliance. Retrieved 24 September 2021, from
https://covid19criticalcare.com/about/the-flccc-physicians/

[87] *I-RECOVER Protocol | FLCCC | Front Line COVID-19 Critical Care Alliance. (2021). Retrieved 24 September 2021, from https://covid19criticalcare.com/covid-19-protocols/i-recover-protocol/*

[88] *Who We Are - IncellDx. (2021). Retrieved 24 September 2021, from https://incelldx.com/who-we-are/*

[89] *A Solution for Longhaulers is Coming Soon. (2020). Retrieved 24 September 2021, from https://covid.us.org/2020/09/21/a-solution-for-longhaulers-is-coming-soon/*

[90] *Chronic COVID Treatment Center™ Retrieved 24 September 2021, from https://covidlonghaulers.com/*

[91] *Doctor Says These Existing drugs Can Help Long COVID | Eat This Not That. (2021). Retrieved 24 September 2021, from https://www.eatthis.com/news-long-covid-cure-doctor-patterson/; Johnson, C. (2021). Has Bruce Patterson Cracked Long COVID? - Health Rising. Retrieved 24 September 2021, from https://www.healthrising.org/blog/2021/07/21/patterson-cracked-long-covid/; Johnson, C. (2021). Has Bruce Patterson Cracked Long COVID? - Health Rising.*

[92] Patterson, B., Guevara-Coto, J., YogenDr.a, R., Francisco, E., Long, E., & Pise, A. et al. (2021). *Immune-Based Prediction of COVID-19 Severity and Chronicity Decoded Using Machine Learning. Frontiers In Immunology, 12.* DOI: 10.3389/fimmu.2021.700782; Patterson, B., Francisco, E., YogenDr.a, R., Long, E., Pise, A., & RoDr.igues, H. et al. (2021). *Persistence of SARS CoV-2 S1 Protein in CD16+ Monocytes in Post-Acute Sequelae of COVID-19 (PASC) Up to 15 Months Post-Infection.* DOI: 10.1101/2021.06.25.449905

[93] Arthur, J., Forrest, J., Boehme, K., Kennedy, J., Owens, S., & Herzog, C. et al. (2021). *Development of ACE2 autoantibodies after SARS-CoV-2 infection. PLOS ONE, 16(9),* e0257016. DOI: 10.1371/journal.pone.0257016

[94] *Some With Long-Haul COVID See Relief After Vaccination.* (2021). Retrieved 24 September 2021, from https://www.webmd.com/vaccines/covid-19-vaccine/news/20210317/some-with-long-haul-covid-see-relief-after-vaccination

[95] Viebahn-Haensler, R., & León Fernández, O. (2021). *Ozone in Medicine. The Low-Dose Ozone Concept and Its Basic Biochemical Mechanisms of Action in Chronic Inflammatory Diseases. International Journal Of Molecular Sciences, 22(15),* 7890. DOI: 10.3390/ijms22157890. *A book by the physician Dr.. David Brownstein explores the use of ozone therapy: Ozone: The Miracle Therapy — Dr. Brownstein's Holistic Medicine.* (2021). Retrieved 24 September 2021, from https://cube-blackbird-rjba.squarespace.com/shop/p/ozone-the-miracle-therapy

[96] Manjunath, S., Sakar, M., Katapadi, M., & Geetha Balakrishna, R. (2021). Recent case studies on the use of ozone to combat coronavirus: Problems and perspectives. Environmental Technology & Innovation, 21, 101313. DOI: 10.1016/j.eti.2020.101313; Hernández, A., Viñals, M., Isidoro, T., & Vilás, F. (2020). Potential Role of Oxygen–Ozone Therapy in Treatment of COVID-19 Pneumonia. American Journal Of Case Reports, 21. DOI: 10.12659/ajcr.925849.

[97] Younger, J., Parkitny, L., & McLain, D. (2014). The use of low-dose naltrexone (LDN) as a novel anti-inflammatory treatment for chronic pain. Clinical Rheumatology, 33(4), 451-459. DOI: 10.1007/s10067-014-2517-2

[98] Pilot Study Into LDN and NAD+ for Treatment of Patients With Post-COVID-19 Syndrome - Full-Text View - ClinicalTrials.gov. (2021). Retrieved 24 September 2021, from https://clinicaltrials.gov/ct2/show/NCT04604704. For more information visit https://ldnresearchtrust.org/about-the-ldn-research-trust

[99] Homeopathy for Post Covid Syndrome - Support & Symptom Management. (2020). Retrieved 24 September 2021, from https://www.Dr.homeo.com/homeopathic-treatment/homeopathy-for-post-covid-syndrome/

[100] *Acupuncture - Mayo Clinic. (2021). Retrieved 24 September 2021, from https://www.mayoclinic.org/tests-procedures/acupuncture/about/pac-20392763*

[101] *Han, Z., Zhang, Y., Wang, P., Tang, Q., & Zhang, K. (2021). Is acupuncture effective in the treatment of COVID-19 related symptoms? Based on bioinformatics/network topology strategy. Briefings In Bioinformatics, 22(5). doi: 10.1093/bib/bbab110*

[102] *The study finds promising results using acupuncture to treat inflammation. (2020). Retrieved 24 September 2021, from https://news.harvard.edu/gazette/story/2020/08/study-reveals-acupuncture-affects-disease-course/*

[103] *Alschuler, L., Chiasson, A., Horwitz, R., Sternberg, E., Crocker, R., Weil, A., & Maizes, V. (2020). Integrative medicine considerations for convalescence from mild-to-moderate COVID-19 disease. EXPLORE. DOI: 10.1016/j.explore.2020.12.005*

[104] *Doctors couldn't help these COVID-19 patients with their endless symptoms. So they turned to one another. (2020). Retrieved 18 September 2021, from https://www.nbcnews.com/health/health-news/doctors-couldn-t-help-these-covid-19-patients-their-endless-n1208116*

GHR

VOL. 01/2021   PUBLISIHING NEWS

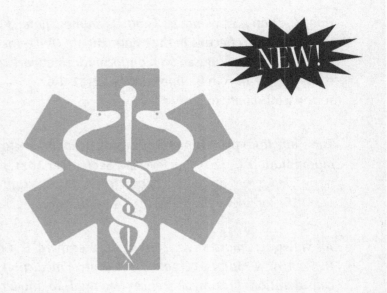

THIRTEEN DIFFERENT MODALITIES INCLUDING LINKS TO THEIR PRACTITIONERS.

A Comprehensive Guide to Non-Conventional Treatments for Chronic Diseases

JDGOODMAN.CA/ROADMAP-TO-RECOVERY

Made in United States
North Haven, CT
21 September 2022

24414088R00095